PERCUTANEOUS BIOPSY, ASPIRATION AND DRAINAGE

Percutaneous Biopsy, Aspiration and Drainage

Janis G. Letourneau, M.D.
Assistant Professor of Radiology
University of Minnesota Medical School
Minneapolis, Minnesota

Morteza K. Elyaderani, M.D.
Professor of Radiology
Creighton University School of Medicine
Director of Invasive Radiology and Ultrasound
St. Joseph Hospital
Omaha, Nebraska

Wilfrido R. Castañeda-Zuñiga, M.D.
Professor, Department of Diagnostic Radiology
University of Minnesota Medical School
Minneapolis, Minnesota

YEAR BOOK MEDICAL PUBLISHERS, INC.
Chicago ● London

Library of Congress Cataloging-in-Publication Data

Letourneau, Janis G.
  Percutaneous biopsy, aspiration and drainage.

  Includes bibliographies and index.
  1. Biopsy, Needle. 2. Drainage, Surgical.
I. Elyaderani, Morteza K.   II. Castañeda-Zuñiga,
Wilfrido R.   III. Title. [DNLM: 1. Biopsy, Needle—
methods. 2. Drainage—methods.   WB 379 C346p]
ISBN 0–8151–1444–3

1 2 3 4 5 6 7 8 9 0 MC 91 90 89 88 87

Sponsoring Editor: James D. Ryan, Jr.
Manager, Copyediting Services: Frances M. Perveiler
Production Project Manager: Etta Worthington
Proofroom Supervisor: Shirley E. Taylor

Contributors

Wilfrido R. Castañeda-Zuñiga, M.D.
Professor, Department of Diagnostic Radiology
University of Minnesota Medical School
Minneapolis, Minnesota

Morteza K. Elyaderani, M.D.
Professor of Radiology
Creighton University School of Medicine
Director of Invasive Radiology and Ultrasound
St. Joseph Hospital
Omaha, Nebraska

Yukiyoshi Kimura, M.D.
Clinica Londres
Clazada Las Aguilas
Mexico

Karen J. Laffey, M.D., Ph.D.
Assistant Professor of Radiology
Columbia University College of Physicians and Surgeons
Assistant Attending Radiologist
Columbia-Presbyterian Medical Center
New York, New York

Janis G. Letourneau, M.D.
Assistant Professor of Radiology
University of Minnesota Medical School
Minneapolis, Minnesota

Eric C. Martin, M.A., (Oxon.), M.R.C.P., F.R.C.R.
Professor of Clinical Radiology
Columbia University College of Physicians and Surgeons
Director of Cardiovascular and Interventional Radiology
Columbia-Presbyterian Medical Center
New York, New York

Preface

Percutaneous radiologic procedures have come of age over recent years. Much of the success of these procedures can be attributed to advances in fluoroscopic and cross-sectional imaging and to advances in instrumentation. In addition, cytologic diagnosis is now readily accepted in many institutions. Aspiration and catheter drainage are also regarded as potentially curative by both radiologists and clinicians. Percutaneous biopsy, aspiration, and drainage represent a significant part of our radiologic practices.

This book is an up-to-date technical guide to percutaneous biopsy, aspiration, and drainage. It discusses localization with fluoroscopy, ultrasound, and computed tomography. It describes biopsy and drainage instrumentation in detail. Regional considerations of biopsy and drainage are made in separate chapters with respect to lesions in the chest, breast, liver, pancreas, kidneys and adrenals, retroperitoneum and pelvis. More detailed analyses of abscess drainage and amniocentesis are included. The accuracy and complications of biopsy and drainage are also discussed.

The goal of this book is to provide a concise, practical guide to biopsy, aspiration, and drainage for the practicing radiologist. A secondary goal is to provide a source of reference for clinicians interested in these procedures.

JANIS G. LETOURNEAU, M.D.

Contents

Preface vii

1 / General Considerations of Percutaneous Biopsy and Drainage
by Janis G. Letourneau and Morteza K. Elyaderani. 1

2 / Fluoroscopy-Guided Biopsy of Chest Masses *by Janis G. Letourneau,
Yukiyoshi Kimura, and Wilfrido R. Castañeda-Zuñiga* 30

3 / Percutaneous Aspiration of Thoracic Fluid Collections
and Masses With Ultrasound Guidance *by Janis G. Letourneau
and Morteza K. Elyaderani*. 40

4 / Percutaneous Aspiration and Drainage of Thoracic Masses
With Computed Tomographic Guidance *by Janis G. Letourneau* . . . 51

5 / Fluoroscopy-Guided Transabdominal Biopsy of Retroperitoneal
Masses *by Janis G. Letourneau, Yukiyoshi Kimura, and Wilfrido R.
Castañeda-Zuñiga* 59

6 / Pancreatic Biopsy and Drainage Guided by Ultrasound
and Computed Tomography *by Janis G. Letourneau
and Morteza K. Elyaderani*. 66

7 / Percutaneous Biopsy of Kidneys and Adrenals and Drainage
of Nephric and Perinephric Fluid Collections *by Janis G. Letourneau
and Morteza K. Elyaderani*. 79

8 / Percutaneous Aspiration and Drainage of the Liver Guided
by Ultrasound and Computed Tomography *by Janis G. Letourneau
and Morteza K. Elyaderani*. 104

9 / Percutaneous Drainage of Abscesses *by Eric C. Martin
and Karen J. Laffey* 121

10 / Percutaneous Biopsy and Drainage of Pelvic Masses
by Janis G. Letourneau 139

11 / Aspirations Performed for Miscellaneous Conditions
by Morteza K. Elyaderani 146

Index 159

1

General Considerations of Percutaneous Biopsy and Drainage

Janis G. Letourneau, M.D.
Morteza K. Elyaderani, M.D.

Fine-needle aspiration biopsy has gained wide acceptance because of its simplicity, safety, and accuracy. In 1930, the pioneers of aspiration biopsy, Martin and Ellis of Memorial Hospital in New York, reported on 65 patients with malignancy confirmed by needle puncture and aspiration.[23] However, the value of the procedure was not appreciated at that time. Newer imaging modalities such as ultrasonography (US) and computed tomography (CT) have contributed to the general popularity of fine-needle aspiration, as they permit more accurate lesion localization. In addition, use of a thin-walled, fine-gauge needle generally assures a safe procedure. With refined techniques and increased experience amongst radiologists and cytologists, the rate of accuracy of fine-needle aspiration biopsy has increased to 80% to 90%, with few complications. Fine-needle aspiration typically yields tissue for cytologic examination, but with technical variations can also yield tissue for histologic examination. Percutaneous biopsy is not limited to the diagnosis of neoplastic processes, as specimens for bacteriologic and chemical analysis may also be sent when appropriate.

The development of percutaneous drainage techniques, both those of simple aspiration and catheter drainage, has paralleled technical advances in aspiration biopsy and other areas of interventional radiology. Similarly, technical developments in US and CT have provided more accurate means of localization than was previously available. Therapeutic drainage is frequently performed in conjunction with diagnostic aspiration, although it can be done as a primary procedure.

LOCALIZATION

Precise localization of the mass or fluid collection is essential for performance of a successful biopsy or drainage. This can be accomplished by a variety of means, but most commonly is accomplished by fluoroscopic, sonographic, or CT guidance. Fluoroscopic guidance can be facilitated by administration of contrast in the vascular system (intravenously or intra-arterially), lymphatic system, or biliary system. This chapter will deal with the topics of sonographic and CT localization for percutaneous biopsy and drainage.

Static and real-time sonography can both be used to localize for percutaneous biopsy and drainage. Both linear-array and sector real-time scanners can be used for these purposes. Real-time sonography is better suited for these tasks, as continuous monitoring of the needle position during placement is possible. In many instances, however, continuous visualization of the needle is not necessary, and static images are then sufficient for localization. Biopsy transducers are available for both static and real-time sonographic units.

In general, the target must be localized in two planes. This is best accomplished with the patient in suspended quiet respiration. It is desirable to align the path of the needle so that it is perpendicular to the skin surface, defining the shortest tract for the needle. This is not always possible, however, because of the presence of intervening structures such as the pleural space or the gallbladder. These circumstances may necessitate the use of an angled course. The depth to the target can be determined electronically using the capabilities of the US unit.

Target localization with a static scanner without a biopsy transducer requires repetitive scanning in longitudinal and transverse planes. When a desirable needle course is identified, the transducer is held intermittently in that location and the electronic marking line is activated. The marking line should be exactly superimposed on the intended course of the needle in two planes (Fig 1–1). Before the transducer is removed from the skin, it can be placed precisely over the intended site of needle entry and angled according to the previous localization to provide a final check with the marking line. The transducer is then removed to allow for preparation of the skin at the site of puncture.

Static US units can be used for localization with a biopsy transducer.[15] Such a transducer has a central canal through which a needle can be placed (Fig 1–2). Initial localization is done with a standard transducer as described above. This transducer is then removed and the skin site is prepared for the procedure. The sterilized biopsy transducer is mounted on the articulated arm of the scanner and the target is rescanned using a sterile coupling agent. The intended needle course is again confirmed using the electronic marking line. The distance from the skin to a target point within the mass plus the length of the biopsy transducer is calculated, and this distance is marked on the needle to be used. With this technique the needle tip is not imaged on the screen.

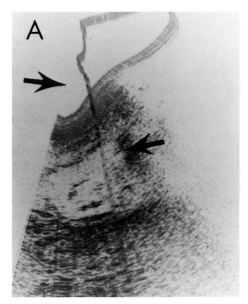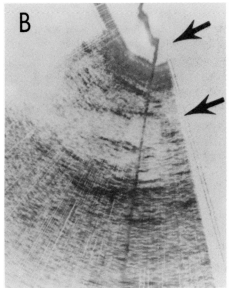

FIG 1–1.
A, transverse and **B,** longitudinal localization of a renal mass *(lower arrows)* by B-mode scanning. Dark line demonstrates the angle of approach *(upper arrows)*.

Once the needle is in position within the target, the biopsy transducer can be removed from the needle through a slit and the remainder of the procedure can be performed without the transducer.

Real-time US units can also be used for localization for percutaneous biopsy or drainage. This can be accomplished without or with a specially de-

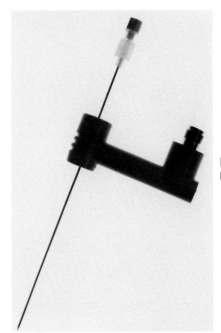

FIG 1–2.
B-mode biopsy transducer with central canal.

signed biopsy transducer or side-arm attachment for the transducer that holds and guides the biopsy needle. Localization of the target in two planes is facilitated with real-time scanning.

Linear-array transducers are constructed from a large number of transducers positioned side-by-side. Their major disadvantage for use in percutaneous procedures is their bulky size, making skin contact sometimes difficult and making manipulations cumbersome. When used without a special biopsy adaptation, a longitudinal scan is made over the region of interest. A 22-gauge needle is then slipped between the transducer and the skin of the patient. The needle casts an acoustic shadow and, by careful repositioning of the needle, the shadow is superimposed on the desired needle tract to the target. This position is then marked on the patient's skin. The procedure is then repeated in the horizontal plane. The intersection of the two needle alignments defines the site of entry of the biopsy needle (Fig 1–3). The depth to the target can be determined electronically from the scanner. The aspirating needle is inserted to the lesion according to the predetermined angle and depth following skin preparation and application of anesthesia. An adaptor for biopsy with linear-array transducers (Fig 1–4) has also been described.[27]

Linear-array biopsy transducers are usually designed with a central canal for needle insertion (Fig 1–5).[26] A small acoustic shadow is produced by the central canal in the center of the image. When this is situated over the target in two planes the needle can be introduced. Other biopsy transducers have a

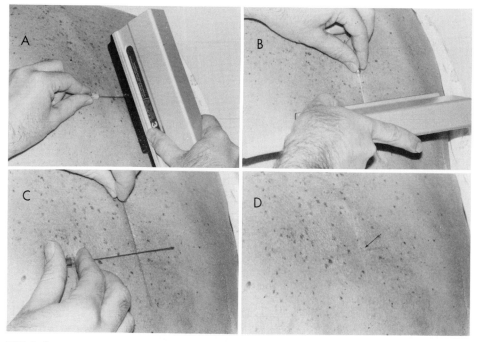

FIG 1–3.
Localization with a linear-array transducer done by slipping a needle between the transducer and the patient's skin. **A,** longitudinal; **B,** transverse; **C,** crossing point of longitudinal and transverse needles; **D,** impression of the needle over the skin *(arrow).*

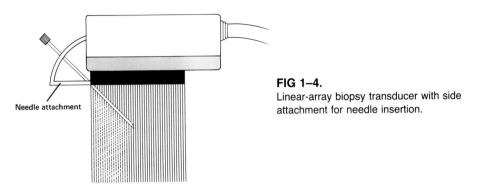

FIG 1–4.
Linear-array biopsy transducer with side attachment for needle insertion.

Needle attachment

snap-on attachment on the center of the transducer that holds the aspiration needle in place once the needle tract has been determined. A small canal between the attachment and the transducer allows the needle to be advanced. These transducers must be sterilized before localization and biopsy. A sterile coupling agent is used. The needle is marked to a distance that includes the depth of the target from the skin surface and the height of the biopsy transducer. The needle is advanced in suspended quiet respiration and its position can be monitored. A fine, 22- or 23-gauge needle may not be easily visible, particularly in a solid mass. The position of its tip may be inferred by the presence of an acoustic shadow.[9] Larger needles are more readily visible. When the needle tip is positioned within the target, the transducer can be removed to facilitate aspiration.

Sector scanners can also be used for aspiration procedures. Their compact size permits good skin coupling and facilitates localization and needle manipulation. Side-arm attachments are available for some transducers.[22, 29] These allow advancement of the needle in the sector plane along different degrees of angulation (Fig 1–6). Side-arm attachments must be sterilized for these procedures and are then attached to a sterile or sheathed transducer. An attachment is also available for phased-array real-time scanning units.[5] Their use is not necessary, as the biopsy needle can be advanced alongside the transducer in the plane of the sector. This allows for continuous visualization of the needle shaft and tip during the procedure. In this latter situation, the transducer must

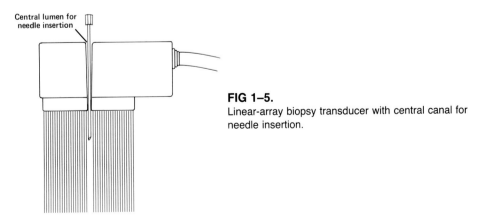

Central lumen for needle insertion

FIG 1–5.
Linear-array biopsy transducer with central canal for needle insertion.

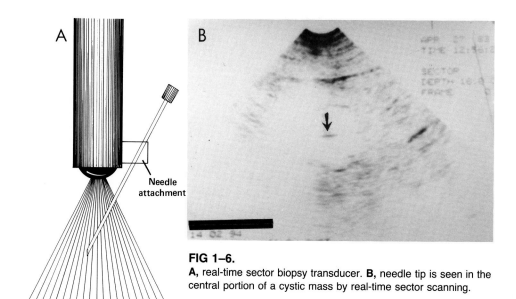

FIG 1–6.
A, real-time sector biopsy transducer. **B,** needle tip is seen in the central portion of a cystic mass by real-time sector scanning.

be sterilized or placed in a sterile glove or sheath coated with an acoustic coupling agent to permit an aseptic procedure.

Localization for percutaneous needle placement with a sector scanner must be done in two perpendicular planes. The target lesion must be situated precisely in the center of the image from these planes of examination. The transducer must also be held at the angle of the intended needle course. This ideally is perpendicular to the skin surface, but this is sometimes not feasible, as mentioned earlier, because of intervening structures.

For all of these methods of localization the patient should be positioned so that the target lesion is most accessible. Planning of intended needle path should also take into account the location of nearby vital structures. When aspiration of freely flowing fluid in the pleural or peritoneal cavities is requested, the patient can be positioned to maximize fluid accumulation in a dependent fashion. Once lesion localization is completed, percutaneous fine-needle biopsy can be performed with a tandem, coaxial, or modified coaxial technique. These techniques are discussed later in this chapter. If the target lesion is superficial in location and distant from vital structures, localization and biopsy can be accomplished with a larger gauge needle.

Computed Tomographic Localization

Computed tomography is also an acceptable means of localization for percutaneous biopsy and drainage. It can be used for localization of lesions in many anatomic regions, including some that are difficult to image by other modalities. It does present some technical limitations. The most compelling of these is one's inability to continuously monitor needle position during placement. More importantly, the needle tip position cannot be confirmed on occasion by repeat scanning, because the location of the lesion, the uninserted length of the needle, and the small diameter of the gantry aperture do not permit repositioning of the patient in the CT scanner gantry.

Diagnostic images are obtained in a transaxial plane. The patient is then placed in the CT scanner gantry in a position that is thought will make the target lesion most accessible. The optimal plane for biopsy is selected (Fig 1–7,A) and a repeat scan is obtained at that level following placement of a grid or marker on the skin over the region of interest[37] (Fig 1–7,B). This permits a more precise definition of the needle tract, should any angulation of the needle be required to avoid intervening structures. Angulation of the intended needle path from the horizontal or parasagittal planes, as well as the depth to the target lesion, can be determined electronically from the CT scanner.

The intended puncture site is marked and prepared. The needle is inserted with the patient in suspended quiet respiration to the predetermined depth and angle. The patient is allowed to resume quiet respiration and the region is rescanned to verify that the needle tip is in the desired location within the target lesion (Fig 1–7,D). Once this verification is obtained the patient is taken out from the scanner gantry and the procedure is completed.

Depending on the location of lesion and location of nearby potentially vital structures, initial localization may be accomplished with either a fine-needle or

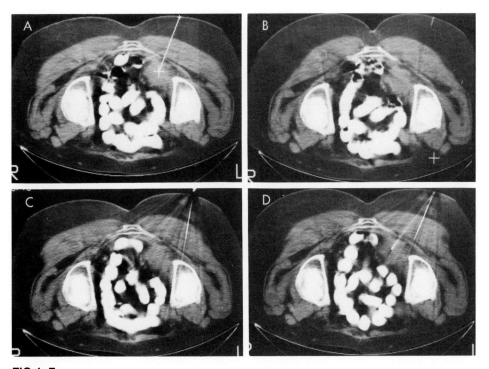

FIG 1–7.
A, computed tomographic image (patient prone) shows a soft-tissue mass in the posterior pelvis. The site of entry and angle of approach are demonstrated. **B,** short 22-gauge needle is inserted at the site of entry and a scan is obtained. **C,** 22-gauge needle is inserted and the scan is repeated. In this figure the needle is not properly directed. **D,** another 22-gauge needle is inserted, with the first needle left in place.

a larger gauge needle. If a fine-needle is chosen for initial localization, biopsy can be performed with a tandem, coaxial, or modified coaxial technique.

As with US localization, it is most desirable to direct the needle course perpendicular to the skin surface. Sometimes, primarily because of location of the pleural reflection, this is not feasible and an angled path must be taken. The angulation of the needle course can be calculated using data relating to the depth of the target lesion and the location of the puncture site (Fig 1–8).[7, 11, 13, 35]

ASPIRATION BIOPSY

Instrumentation

Biopsy Needles
Several kinds of biopsy needles are commercially available, including aspiration, cutting, and screw-type needles. In general, they range in size from 23- to 16-gauge and from 10 to 20 cm in length. It was established long ago in relation to thoracic biopsy that fine-needles are associated with lower incidence of complications[38]; however, the flexibility of thin-walled, fine-caliber needles sometimes makes them difficult to control during placement (Fig 1–9).

The 22- and 23-gauge Chiba needles are frequently used for aspiration biopsy. These have a sharp 25°, beveled tip and inner stylet that prevents tissue from entering the lumen during placement (Fig 1–10). They are primarily used for obtaining cytologic and bacteriologic material, although histologic cores also can be obtained with their use. The Turner needle, available in 16-, 18-, 20-, and 22-gauges, is similar to the Chiba needle, but has a 45° bevel[31] (Fig 1–11). It is thought that the steeper bevel angle makes it easier to obtain a core of tissue for histologic examination.[21]

Many needles have been designed to enhance tissue coring by use of a cutting tip; several of these are also available in fine caliber. The Greene needle

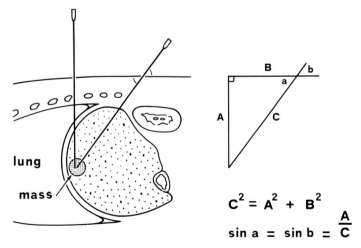

FIG 1–8.
Technique of triangulation fine-needle aspiration by computed tomography.

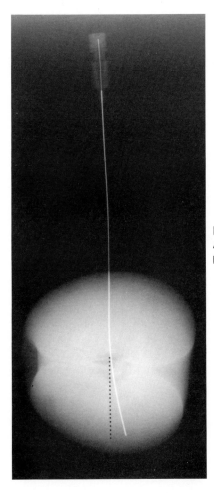

FIG 1–9.
A fine needle bends due to tissue resistance or deep position of target lesion.

is a modified fine-needle (22- and 23-gauge) with a circumferentially sharpened tip that allows the aspiration of a tissue core by means of a rotary movement.[17] The Sure-cut is another cutting needle that is available for aspiration biopsy in 19-, 21- and 22-gauges, as well as in the larger 15-, 16-, 17-, and 18-gauge calibers (Fig 1–12). The Franseen needle, available in 18-, 20-, and 22-gauges, has three cutting serrations that also produce a tissue core or fragments when the needle is rotated[2, 3, 8] (Fig 1–13). The 20-gauge Westcott needle has a slotted tip for obtaining a tissue core[36] (Fig 1–14). The larger 17-gauge Lee needle has a cutting tip and an inner needle fashioned with a biopsy window. It is effective in obtaining histologic specimens.[20] These larger needles, and the even larger 14-gauge Tru-cut needles[12] with a 2-cm long specimen window (Fig 1–15), are recommended for use only when biopsy can be accomplished with the needle coursing through no vital structures or bowel.

Sets for facilitating biopsy with the coaxial technique are also commercially available. These include the Greene biopsy set (Cook, Inc.; Medi-tech, Inc.) with a larger spinal needle for placement and a fine Greene needle for biopsy[10] (Fig 1–16). The vanSonnenberg biopsy set (Cook, Inc.) is also available. It has

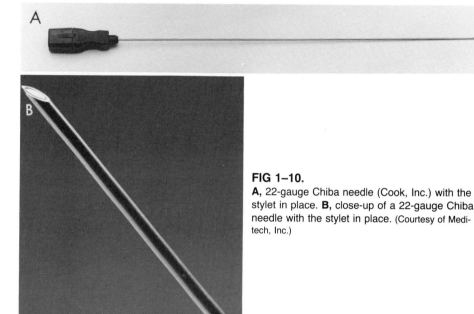

FIG 1–10.
A, 22-gauge Chiba needle (Cook, Inc.) with the stylet in place. **B,** close-up of a 22-gauge Chiba needle with the stylet in place. (Courtesy of Meditech, Inc.)

a fine-needle with a detachable hub for initial placement and a stabilizing larger needle that slides over the needle with a detachable hub. The larger needle provides a guide for repeated fine-needle aspiration biopsy[34] (Fig 1–17).

The Rotex biopsy instrument is a screw-type needle.[25] It consists of a 160-mm long outer cannula that is 1.0 mm in diameter and has a cutting edge at its tip. A screw-tipped stylet, 0.55 mm in diameter and 195 mm in length, is inserted into the outer cannula. Tissue sampling is done with the distal 15 mm of the inner stylet as it is advanced into the lesion. Good diagnostic results have been obtained with this needle in the biopsy of both benign and malignant lesions.[16]

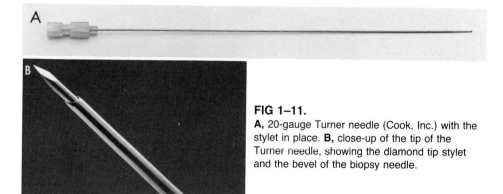

FIG 1–11.
A, 20-gauge Turner needle (Cook, Inc.) with the stylet in place. **B,** close-up of the tip of the Turner needle, showing the diamond tip stylet and the bevel of the biopsy needle.

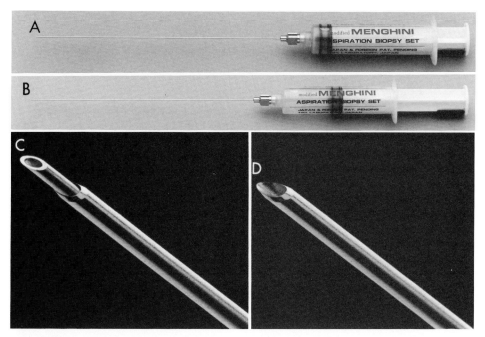

FIG 1–12.
A, 21-gauge Sure-Cut aspiration biopsy set with the plunger of the syringe in place for needle advancement. **B,** the biopsy set with the plunger of the syringe retracted for biopsy. **C,** close-up of the needle tip with the stylet protruding as it does with the syringe plunger in. **D,** close-up of the needle with the stylet retracted for biopsy.

Technique

Percutaneous biopsy can be performed as an inpatient or outpatient procedure following the procural of informed consent. Patient preparation will depend in large part on the imaging modality intended for use in localization. Fasting from midnight will be useful in those patients who undergo localization of the lesion with fluoroscopy if contrast material is to be administered, particularly

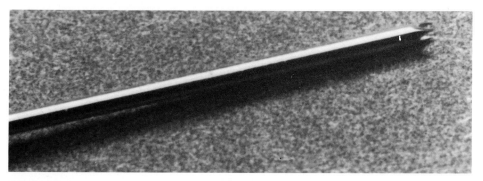

FIG 1–13.
Close-up view of the serrated tip of a Franseen-type needle (Crown biopsy needle; Medi-tech, Inc.) (Courtesy of Medi-tech, Inc.)

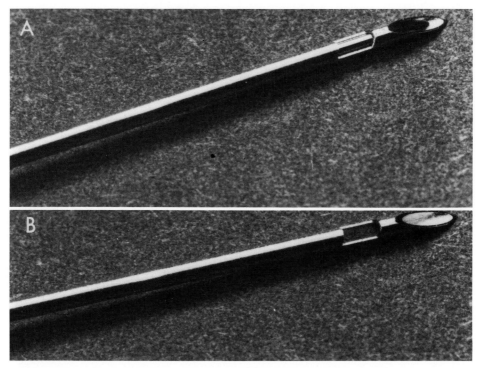

FIG 1–14.
A, closed tip of a 20-gauge Westcott-type needle (Notched biopsy needle; Medi-tech, Inc.). **B,** tip of the same needle with the biopsy window exposed by withdrawal of the stylet. (Courtesy of Medi-tech, Inc.)

intravenous (IV) contrast, or in those who undergo localization with US, as ingestion of both liquids and solids is associated with the presence of intestinal gas, which can obscure underlying abdominal structures. With CT localization, fasting may also be indicated if use of IV contrast is planned. Bowel opacification with oral or rectal contrast may also be of value with CT localization.

A minimum of laboratory testing is necessary before most aspiration biopsies. This should include a complete blood cell (CBC) count with platelet quantification, and partial thromboplastin and prothrombin times. If possible, abnormal bleeding parameters should be corrected before the procedure, especially if a large gauge needle will be used for biopsy. Adequate renal function should be documented with determinations of blood urea nitrogen and creatinine in those patients who will receive IV contrast material.

Use of premedication is not necessary in most patients. However, the procedure will often be facilitated if pediatric and apprehensive adult patients are treated before the procedure. A relaxant or analgesic can be administered during the procedure if necessary. Antibiotics may be given before biopsy or drainage of any lesion suspected to be infected.

Most patients will be candidates for percutaneous biopsy. Some degree of patient cooperation is valuable, however, to allow for accurate lesion localiza-

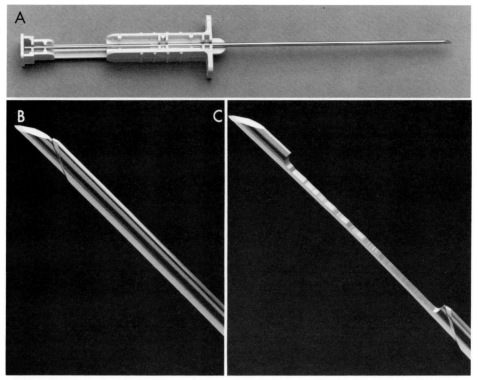

FIG 1–15.
A, Tru-cut needle (Travenol, Inc.) showing handle apparatus that retracts the cannula, exposing the biopsy window. **B,** needle tip with the outer cannula covering the large biopsy notch. **C,** retraction of the outer cannula reveals the 2 cm biopsy window.

tion and to permit precise needle placement. Consequently, aspiration biopsy may be contraindicated in agitated and uncooperative patients or in those with an uncontrollable cough. Suspected echinococcal cysts should not be aspirated because of the risks of seeding daughter cysts and generalized anaphylaxis.[28]

Once the lesion has been localized and the puncture site is chosen, the skin is marked and cleansed with antiseptic solution. Sterile drapes are placed around the puncture site. Local anesthesia is administered. Needle placement is usually facilitated by producing a small nick in the skin with a scalpel blade. Needle placement should be performed with the patient in suspended respiration (Fig 1–18). With fluoroscopic and US guidance the biopsy needle is advanced to the margin of the lesion in small increments using continuous visualization. With CT guidance the needle is advanced in a single smooth motion to the desired depth and the patient is then allowed to breathe quietly while a repeat scan is taken at the level of the needle to verify the needle tip position.

The optimal position for the aspirating needle tip will vary slightly depending on the radiographic features of the lesion. If possible, a more solid or potentially neoplastic lesion is biopsied at its margin. A more cystic or potentially infected mass is better aspirated near its center.

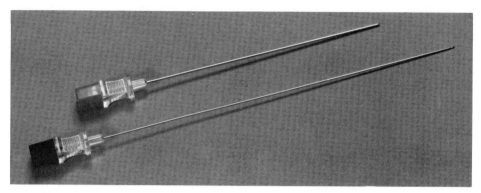

FIG 1–16.
Greene-type coaxial biopsy set (Co-axial lung biopsy set; Medi-tech, Inc.) features a larger localization needle and a fine biopsy needle. The set can be used for biopsies in extrathoracic locations. (Courtesy of Medi-tech, Inc.)

Actual aspiration biopsy can be accomplished in a variety of ways. Multiple independent passes with the biopsy needle along the designated needle tract can be made with minor changes in the angulation of the needle to sample different areas of the target lesion. This should be done only with fine-needles unless the target lesion is situated superficially. A tandem technique can be used[7] to facilitate the biopsy procedure. A fine-needle is placed initially in the lesion and is used as a guide for multiple passes with a second biopsy needle. The second needle is passed along the side of the guiding needle with slight variations in the needle angulation made if desired. A coaxial technique[10] also optimizes accurate needle placement. With this method an 18- or 19-gauge guiding needle is used to localize the lesion. A fine-biopsy needle is then passed through the lumen of the larger needle for multiple aspirations. With the modified coaxial technique described by vanSonnenberg et al.[33] and McGahan,[24] initial localization can be made with a fine-needle. The hub can then be cut or removed (if detachable) to allow the placement of a larger needle over it. Multiple biopsy passes can then be made through the lumen of the larger needle once it is fixed in place.

Simple aspiration biopsy is usually accomplished with a needle such as the Chiba or Turner type. Typically, cytologic and bacteriologic samples are obtained with this technique, although histologic samples can also be obtained. For a solid lesion, the needle tip is advanced to the margin of the target with the stylet of the needle in place. The stylet is removed and a polyethylene connecting tube is attached to the needle hub to allow for continuous suction with a 12-ml syringe (Fig 1–19). The needle is then advanced and moved back and forth slightly as it is rotated to obtain the tissue sample. The needle is withdrawn as mild suction is maintained (Figs 1–20 and 21). For a cystic lesion, the center of the lesion is entered and aspiration is accomplished with simple suction.

Biopsy with cutting needles is usually accomplished with a rotary coring motion. Suction is applied to the needle through connecting tubing during final advancement of the needle and during its withdrawal. For those needles

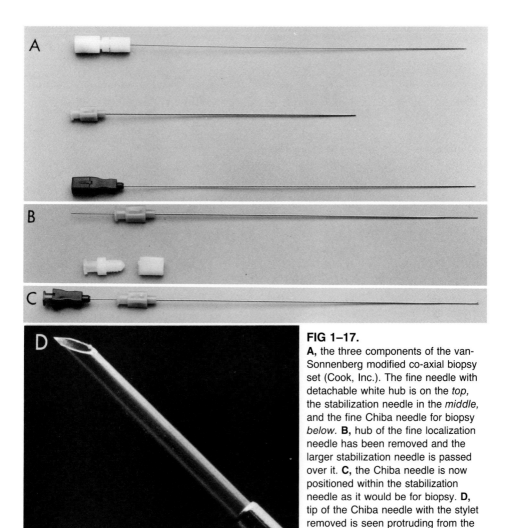

FIG 1-17.
A, the three components of the van-Sonnenberg modified co-axial biopsy set (Cook, Inc.). The fine needle with detachable white hub is on the *top,* the stabilization needle in the *middle,* and the fine Chiba needle for biopsy *below.* **B,** hub of the fine localization needle has been removed and the larger stabilization needle is passed over it. **C,** the Chiba needle is now positioned within the stabilization needle as it would be for biopsy. **D,** tip of the Chiba needle with the stylet removed is seen protruding from the larger stabilization needle.

with a biopsy notch on the inner obturator, biopsy is accomplished by advancing the obturator from the outer cannula and then sliding the outer cannula over the obturator. For biopsy with the Westcott needle, the needle tip is advanced to the periphery of the lesion. The stylet is withdrawn 2 to 3 cm to expose the biopsy slot and the needle is advanced into the lesion. The stylet is removed and suction is applied as the needle is moved back and forth and then withdrawn.[36]

Biopsy using the Rotex needle system is limited to primarily solid lesions. Biopsy with the Rotex instrument is initiated with insertion of the cannula and inner biopsy needle to the margin of the lesion. A screw tip is fashioned on the distal aspect of the inner stylet. As this screw tip is advanced into the lesion, biopsy tissue is fixed onto the instrument. The outer cannula is slid over the screw tip inner stylet, cutting and separating the biopsy specimen from the

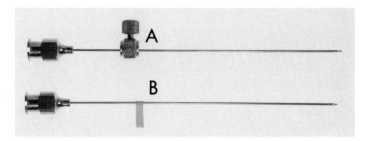

FIG 1–18.
Marking of the designated distance by **(A)** the needle stop or **(B)** Steri-Strip.

remainder of the target lesion. The entire needle system is removed and the biopsy specimen fixed on the distal tip of the inner needle (Fig 1–22).[25] The biopsy specimen must be carefully removed from the screw tip portion of the needle if it does not spontaneously extract itself, with a straight needle or by rolling the needle tip on a glass slide.

Dry or wet aspiration can be performed. Dry aspiration is accomplished without any fluid in the aspirating syringe. Wet aspiration is performed with 1 to 2 ml of sterile nonbacteriostatic saline in the syringe. This has been advocated by some over the traditional dry aspiration technique[17, 37] and can be used with a simple aspirating or cutting-type needle.

Examination of the Aspirated Material

Laboratory examination of the aspirated material will depend in large part on the clinical setting. Cytologic and bacteriologic specimens are routinely obtained. Chemical and cellular analyses will be of value in determining the na-

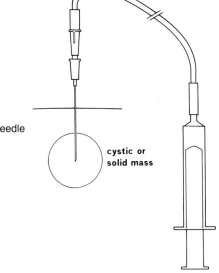

FIG 1–19.
Flexible system provides complete freedom of needle movement during aspiration.

cystic or
solid mass

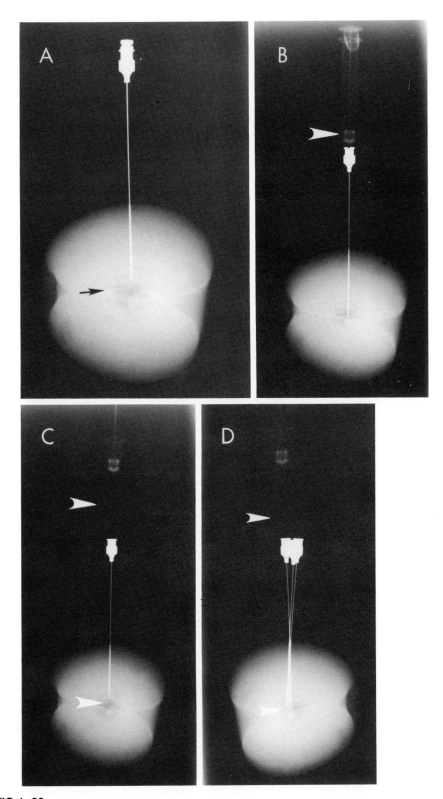

FIG 1–20.
A, the needle tip *(arrow)* is in the margin of the mass (central portion of an apple). **B,** the stylet of the needle is removed and a syringe *(arrowhead)* is connected to the needle. **C,** a vacuum is produced by the syringe. **D,** the needle is advanced and rotated into the target lesion *(lower arrowhead)*.

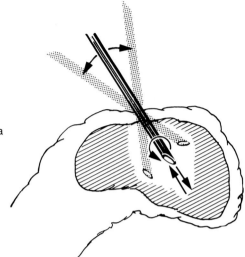

FIG 1–21.
Rotation and advancement of the needle in a
pancreatic mass.

ture of many fluid collections. Depending on the differential diagnosis of the
lesion, lactose dehydrogenase, protein, and bilirubin values may be ordered.
Cell counts can also be obtained.

Microbiologic studies should be ordered in conjunction with the ordering
physician. They frequently include Gram's stain, routine, anaerobic, mycobac-
terial, fungal cultures, and, occasionally, viral cultures.

Cytologic preparations are facilitated by the presence of the cytologist at
the procedure. Once the needle has been removed from the target lesion, the
aspirated material can be expelled for cytologic examination. The material is
expelled onto a glass slide coated with albumin. Multiple expulsions may be
necessary to remove all of the material from the syringe and needle. The aspirate is spread by a second glass slide, making an attempt to separate and

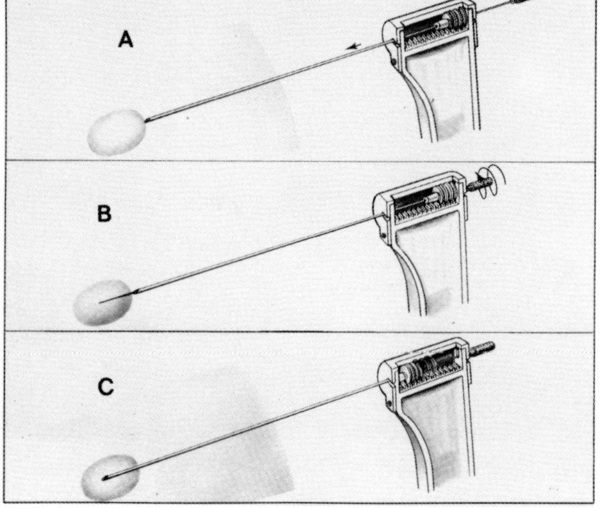

FIG 1–22.
Technique of aspiration by Rotex II
screw-needle. (Courtesy of Bjorn
Nordenstrom, M.D., Professor of
Diagnostic Radiology, Karolinska
Institutet, Sweden.)

A

B

C

distribute cell clumps and tissue fragments. The prepared slides are promptly placed in 95% alcohol (Fig 1–23). Air drying of the slide preparations degrades fixation and nuclear staining. The method of rapid fixation in 95% alcohol preserves nuclear details, so that optimal resemblance between aspirated material and the target lesion is obtained.[18, 30] Ethanol fixation can be prolonged without harm to the specimen for 24 hours if transportation to a distant laboratory is necessary.[19] Alternatively, air-dried smears can be stained according to the May-Grünwald-Giesma method.

Fluid from the aspirate can also be centrifuged. The sediment can then be spread on albumin-coated slides or examined as a cell block by the pathologists. This technique is suitable for aspirates with tiny fragments of tissue and for bloody specimens.

A membrane filtration technique can be used for cytologic preparation as well. A plastic specimen cup is filled with 5 to 10 ml of sterile nonbacteriostatic saline. The contents of the syringe and needle are flushed multiple times with the saline and the suspension is processed as a filter preparation (Fig 1–24). (A cell block could also be prepared if the suspension is thick, bloody, or particulate.) As a filter preparation the material is suctioned into a 5-µ cellulose filter, the supernatant fixed in 95% alcohol, and stained with Papanicolaou's stain.

Any relatively large pieces of aspirated tissue obtained with fine or larger gauge needles should be examined histologically. These fragments require immediate fixation in formalin (Fig 1–25).

DRAINAGE OF FLUID COLLECTIONS

Simple Aspiration

Simple aspiration of fluid collections may result in resolution of the lesion or regression of the patient's symptoms. An attempt at simple aspiration with a needle or needle-sheath system may at times obviate catheter drainage or even an open surgical drainage.

Instrumentation

If fluid is encountered with a percutaneous aspiration, complete evacuation of the fluid collection can be accomplished with the aspirating needle. Some fluid will prove to be too viscous for a fine-needle, such as a 22- or 23-gauge Chiba needle, and complete evacuation of the fluid collection will require placement of a different needle sheath or catheter. Use of a Mitty-Pollack (Cook Urologic, Inc.)[4] coaxial needle for the initial aspiration obviates the need to change from a fine to larger gauge needle (Fig 1–26).

Many different types of needle-sheath systems are commercially available that are suitable for simple aspiration of fluid collections. The Amplatz (Cook, Inc.) angiographic needle set with the stylet and needle removed can be used for aspiration of relatively superficial fluid collections (Fig 1–27). A translumbar aortography needle and sheath set can also be used for deeper collections, using the sheath for aspiration following removal of the stiffening stylet (Fig 1–28).

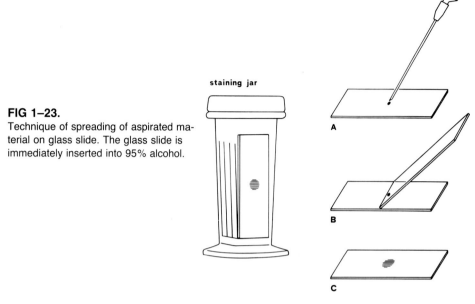

FIG 1–23.
Technique of spreading of aspirated material on glass slide. The glass slide is immediately inserted into 95% alcohol.

For simple aspiration of fluid collections localization must be accurate, and it can be accomplished with fluoroscopy, US, or CT. Depth of the lesion from the skin should be measured electronically with the equipment if possible. Once the lesion is localized, the skin is sterilized and local anesthesia is administered. With fluoroscopy and US, needle or sheath tip position, as well as fluid aspiration, can be monitored continuously. Computed tomographic guidance for such a procedure requires rescanning to document adequate evacuation.

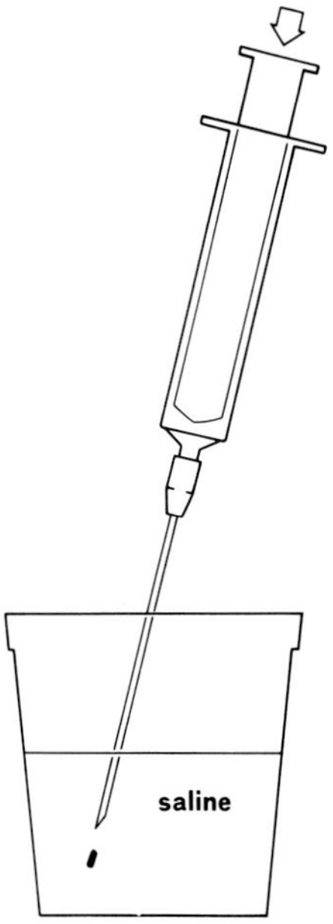

FIG 1–24.
Technique of washing fine needle in a container with saline.

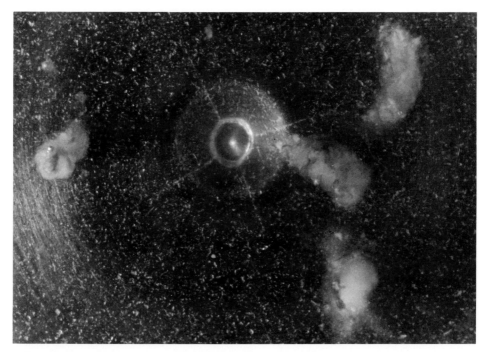

FIG 1–25.
Large fragments of tissue aspirated by fine needle have been placed in formalin.

Catheter Drainage

Depending on their location within the body and their depth, fluid collections can be drained by one of two methods: trocar and Seldinger techniques.

Trocar Technique

The trocar technique is used preferably in patients with fluid collections localized superficially near the abdominal wall without intervening loops of bowel along the needle tract. Guidance methods include fluoroscopy, US, and CT. Ultrasonography and CT can be used either as the sole guidance method for the procedure or to guide the placement of a fine-needle into the abscess, through which contrast medium can be introduced. Subsequently, the place-

FIG 1–26.
The Mitty-Pollack needle set (Cook Urologic, Inc.) includes an 18-gauge needle back-loaded and twist-locked onto a longer 22-gauge needle.

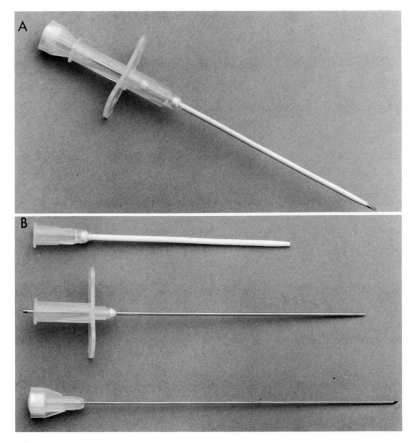

FIG 1–27.
A, an assembled Amplatz arteriotomy set (Cook, Inc.) **B,** components of the Amplatz needle-sheath arteriotomy system. The sheath is on top, the needle in the middle and the stylet below. Once initial placement of the needle-sheath set is accomplished, aspiration or guidewire insertion can be done through the sheath.

ment of the trocar drainage catheter can be accomplished under fluoroscopic control.

Several trocar systems are available commercially; among them is the Hawkins accordion catheter (Cook, Inc.)[14] (Fig 1–29). This system consists of a 45-cm long 22-gauge needle with a 6-F accordion Teflon catheter mounted over the 22-gauge needle and a coat-hanger 0.018-in. guidewire for manipulations. With this system the abscess system is initially punctured with the 22-gauge needle through which contrast medium is injected to document the position of the needle tip within the fluid collection. The 0.018-in. guidewire is then passed through the 22-gauge needle and is looped within the abscess cavity. Holding the wire and the needle stationary, the 6-F Teflon accordion catheter is advanced into the abscess. When a sufficient length of catheter is in the abscess space, the 22-gauge needle and the 0.018-in. guidewire are removed. The accordion catheter loops are tightened by pulling on the monofilament thread, which is then secured to the Luer-Lok side arm adapter. The main advantages of this system are a one-stick introduction and the self-retaining

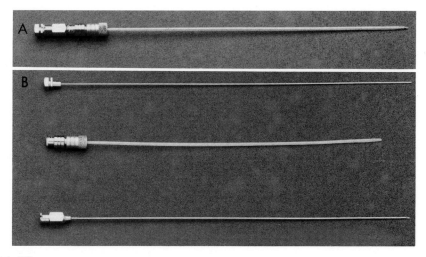

FIG 1–28.
A, assembled translumbar aortography (TLA) needle-sheath set. **B,** disassembled TLA set shows the sheath between the stylet above and the needle below.

properties of the accordion catheter. Its main disadvantage is the small size of the drainage catheter.

The All-purpose Drainage Catheter (Medi-tech, Inc.) is an 8-F catheter system with multiple sideholes in the distal portion of the catheter and a trocar for introduction in one step (Fig 1–30). The Percu-flex material, out of which this catheter is constructed, is comfortable for the patient. Additionally, the large lumen provided by the thin wall of the catheter material facilitates evacuation of purulent material.

The vanSonnenberg sump catheter (Medi-tech, Inc.), constructed of Percu-

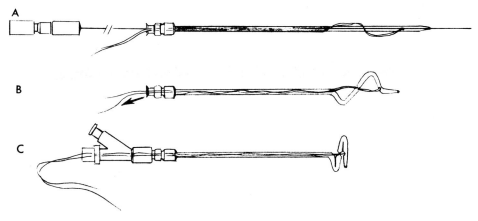

FIG 1–29.
A, the Hawkins accordian needle and catheter system (Cook, Inc.) with the 6 French accordian catheter back-loaded onto a 10 inch 22-gauge needle. Here the catheter has been advanced along the needle, disengaging it from the hub as it would be done following initial puncture of a fluid collection. **B,** the 22-gauge needle has been removed and the accordian tip is formed by retracting the monofilament thread. **C,** the accordian tip is secured by a device in the Luer-Lok hub of the catheter system.

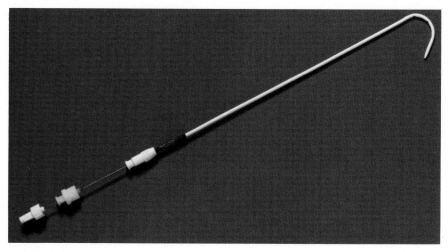

FIG 1–30.
All-purpose drainage catheter with trocar and needle partly loaded (APD catheter; Medi-tech, Inc.)
(Courtesy of Medi-tech, Inc.)

flex, is available in 12 and 14 F (Fig 1–31). This catheter has two lumens, a large one for drainage and a smaller one to act as a sump during drainage. The sump lumen can also be used for the infusion of irrigating fluids and/or antibiotics. The large holes on the inner aspect of the terminal curve of the catheter provide for good drainage. A microbial air filter on the sump ensures sterility through this lumen. A trocar stylet is provided for introduction in one step.[32]

The McLean sump catheter (Cook, Inc.) is similar to the vanSonnenberg system. This C-flex drainage catheter is made in 12- and 16-F sizes and also has two lumens: one for drainage and one for infusion and/or sump purposes. The inner lumen of this catheter is smaller than that of the vanSonnenberg, as the C-flex material is thicker than the Percu-flex material. The McLean catheter also comes with a trocar for introduction in one step. Both of these sump catheters can also be introduced using the Seldinger technique.

Seldinger Technique

The Seldinger angiographic technique can be applied to the drainage of fluid collections. This technique is particularly suitable for fluid collections that are situated deep to the skin or for those that present a difficult approach. Two variations of the technique can be used: a single-stick technique described by Cope and Hawkins and a two-stick technique.

With the Cope single-stick system (Cook, Inc.; Medi-tech, Inc.) a 22-gauge needle is used for the initial puncture of the fluid collection[6] (Fig 1–32). A 0.018-in. guidewire is introduced through the 22-gauge needle and the needle is withdrawn. A dilator, mounted over a 22-gauge cannula, is passed over the 0.018-in. guidewire. Both the dilator and cannula are advanced until the dilator is seen within the abscess cavity. The stiffening cannula and 0.018-in. guidewire are then removed and a 0.038-in. guidewire with a 15-mm "J" is

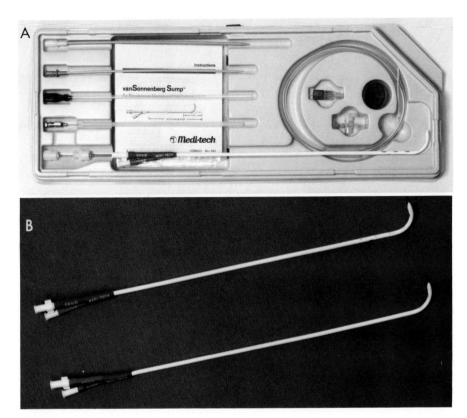

FIG 1–31.
A, vanSonnenberg sump catheter set (Medi-tech, Inc.). **B,** the 2-hole *(below)* and 5-hole varieties *(above)* of vanSonnenberg sump catheters. (Courtesy of Medi-tech, Inc.)

introduced. The wire exits through a sidehole in the dilator into the fluid collection. The dilator is then subsequently removed, leaving the wire in place. Dilation of the tract and placement of the drainage catheter can then be accomplished using the 0.038-in. guidewire. The Hawkins single-stick technique (Cook, Inc.) has been described earlier in discussion of trocar systems. It provides drainage through a 6-F accordion catheter.

The Mitty-Pollack coaxial needle (Cook Urologic, Inc.) is also a single-stick system consisting of a 14-cm long 18-gauge needle mounted over a 22-gauge stylet that measures 22.5 cm (see Fig 1–26). The initial puncture is performed with the 22-gauge component of the needle. Once its position within the fluid collection is documented by the withdrawal of fluid or by the injection of contrast medium, the 18-gauge component of the coaxial needle is advanced over the 22-gauge needle until its tip is situated within the fluid collection. The 22-gauge needle is then withdrawn and a 0.038-in. guidewire can be introduced for dilation of the tract and drainage catheter placement.[4]

The One-Step Insertion needle (Surgitek, Inc.) consists of a 22-gauge stylet over which a 19-gauge needle and a plastic sheath are mounted (Fig 1–33). The initial puncture is done with only the 22-gauge component of the system. Once this is situated within the fluid collection, the 19-gauge needle and plastic

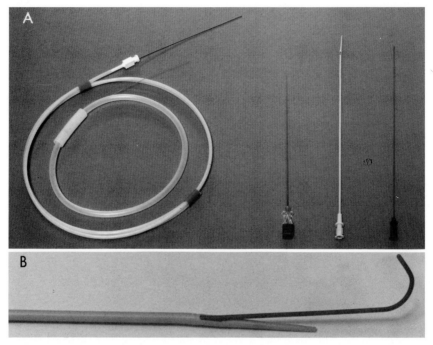

FIG 1–32.
A, components of the one-stick system available through Medi-tech, Inc. Note the two different caliber guidewires, the fine localizing needle, the dilator, and the stiffening cannula. **B,** the dilator tip with the inner stiffening cannula in place. (Courtesy of Medi-tech, Inc.)

sheath are advanced simultaneously. The 22- and 19-gauge needles are then withdrawn, leaving the plastic sheath within the fluid collection for drainage or for introduction of a guidewire, allowing subsequent tract dilation and catheter drainage.

With the two-stick variation of the Seldinger technique, the initial puncture of the fluid collection is performed with a 22-gauge needle. If fluoroscopy is being used to guide the procedure, contrast medium can then be injected to opacify the space. A second puncture is performed with an 18-gauge needle, such as a translumbar aortography sheathed needle, a nephrostomy needle, or an Amplatz arteriotomy needle-sheath system (Cook, Inc.). If fluoroscopic guidance is not being used for catheter placement, the second puncture with the larger needle can be performed in tandem with the fine localizing needle. Use of the Amplatz needle-sheath set is particularly useful when superficially located fluid collections are drained under CT guidance, as the needle will usually fit within the gantry aperature for repeat scanning to document adequate localization.

CONCLUSION

Several basic principles can be applied to percutaneous biopsy and drainage. Accurate localization is of paramount importance. This can be accomplished with fluoroscopy, US, and CT, each method having its advantages and disad-

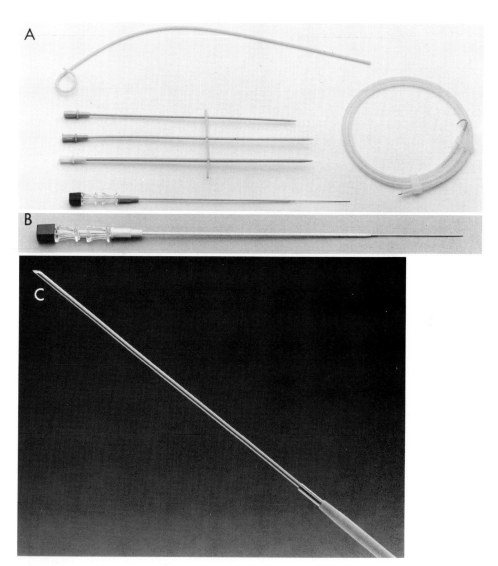

FIG 1–33.
A, components of another single-stick system (One-Step Insertion Set; Surgitek, Inc.). A pigtail catheter, dilators, needle-sheath set and one guidewire are included. **B,** the plastic sheath and 19-gauge needle are back-loaded onto a 22-gauge needle. **C,** close-up of the tip of the needle-sheath elements of the system.

vantages. Many instrumentation systems are available, and familiarity with these systems technically facilitates the performance of biopsy and drainage procedures.

REFERENCES

1. Ackerman LV, Wheat MW: The implantation of cancer. *Surgery* 1955; 37:341.
2. Arnston TL, Boyd WR: Percutaneous biopsy using a safe effective needle. *Radiology* 1978; 127:265.

3. Ballard GL, Boyd WE: A specially designed cutting aspiration needle for lung biopsy. *AJR* 1978; 130:899–903.

4. Baltaxe HA, Mitty HA, Pollack HM: Multipurpose coaxial needle used for percutaneous nephrostomy. *Radiology* 1984; 153:259.

5. Buonocore E, Skipper GJ: Steerable real-time sonographically guided needle biopsy. *AJR* 1981; 136:387–392.

6. Cope C: Conversion from small (0.018") to large (0.038") guidewire in percutaneous drainage procedures. *AJR* 1982; 138:170–171.

7. Ferrucci JT Jr, Wittenberg J: CT biopsy of abdominal tumors: Aids for lesion localization. *Radiology* 1978; 129:739–744.

8. Franseen CC: Aspiration biopsy with a description of a new type of needle. *N Engl J Med* 1941; 224:1054–1055.

9. Goldberg BB, et al: Real-time aspiration-biopsy transducer. *J Clin Ultrasound* 1980; 8:107–112.

10. Greene RF: Transthoracic needle aspiration, in Athanasoulis CA, et al (eds): *Interventional Radiology*. Philadelphia, WB Saunders Co, 1982, pp. 587–634.

11. Haaga JR: New techniques for CT-guided biopsies. *AJR* 1979; 133:633–641.

12. Haaga JR, et al: Clinical comparison of small and large caliber cutting needles for biopsy. *Radiology* 1983; 146:665–667.

13. Haaga JR, et al: CT-guided biopsy. *Cleve Clin Q* 1977; 44:27–33.

14. Hawkins IF: Single-step placement of self-retaining "accordion" catheter. *Semin Interven Radiol* 1984; 1:15–18.

15. Holm HH, Rasmussen SN, Kristensen JK: Ultrasonically guided percutaneous puncture technique. *J Clin Ultrasound* 1973; 1:27–31.

16. House AJS, Thomson KR: Evaluation of a new transthoracic needle for benign and malignant lung lesions. *AJR* 1977; 129:215–220.

17. Isler RJ, et al: Tissue core biopsy of abdominal tumors with a 22-gauge cutting needle. *AJR* 1981; 136:725–728.

18. Jacobsen GK: Aspiration biopsy cytology, in Holm HH, Kristensen JK (eds): *Ultrasonically Guided Puncture Technique*. Philadelphia, WB Saunders Co, 1980.

19. Kline TS: *Handbook of Fine-needle Aspiration Biopsy Cytology*. St Louis, CV Mosby Co, 1981, pp. 1–7.

20. Lee LH: A new biopsy needle and its clinical use. *AJR* 1974; 121:854–859.

21. Lieberman RP, Hafaz GR, Crummy AB: Histology from aspiration biopsy: Turner needle experience. *AJR* 1982; 138:561–564.

22. Lindgren PG: Ultrasonically guided puncture. *Radiology* 1980; 137:235–237.

23. Martin HE, Ellis EB: Biopsy by needle puncture and aspiration. *Ann Surg* 1930; 92:169–191.

24. McGahan JP: Percutaneous biopsy and drainage procedures in the abdomen using a modified coaxial technique. *Radiology* 1984; 153:257–258.

25. Nordenstrom B: A new instrument for biopsy. *Radiology* 1975; 117:474–475.

26. Ohto M, et al: Ultrasonically guided percutaneous contrast medium injection and aspiration biopsy using a real-time puncture transducer. *Radiology* 1980; 136:171–176.

27. Pedersen JF: Percutaneous puncture guided by ultrasonic multitransducer scanning. *J Clin Ultrasound* 1976; 5:175–177.

28. Saidi F: *Surgery of Hydatid Disease*. Philadelphia, WB Saunders Co, 1976.

29. Saitoh M, et al: Ultrasonic real-time guidance for percutaneous puncture. *J Clin Ultrasound* 1979; 7:269–272.

30. Soost HJ: Requirements in gaining and treating biopsy material, in Anacker H, Gullotta U, Rupp N (eds): *Percutaneous Biopsy and Therapeutic Vascular Occlusion*. New York, Thieme-Stratton Inc, 1980.

31. Turner AF, Sargent EN: Percutaneous pulmonary needle biopsy. *AJR* 1968; 104:846–850.

32. vanSonnenberg E: Sump catheter for percutaneous abscess and fluid drainage by trocar or Seldinger technique. *AJR* 1982; 139:613–614.

33. vanSonnenberg E, et al: Percutaneous biopsy of difficult mediastinal, hilar and pulmonary lesions by computed tomographic guidance and a modified coaxial technique. *Radiology* 1983; 148:300–302.

34. vanSonnenberg E, et al: Removable hub needle system for coaxial biopsy of small and difficult lesions. *Radiology* 1984; 152:226.

35. vanSonnenberg E, et al: Triangulation method for percutaneous needle guidance: The angled approach to upper abdominal masses. *AJR* 1981; 137:757–761.

36. Westcott JL: Direct percutaneous needle aspiration of localized pulmonary lesions: Results in 422 patients. *Radiology* 1980; 137:31–35.

37. Wittenberg J, et al: Percutaneous core biopsy of abdominal tumors using 22-gauge needle: Further observations. *AJR* 1982; 139:75–80.

38. Woolf CR: Applications of aspiration lung biopsy with review of the literature. *Dis Chest* 1954; 25:286–300.

2

Fluoroscopy-Guided Biopsy of Chest Masses

Janis G. Letourneau, M.D.
Yukiyoshi Kimura, M.D.
Wilfrido R. Castañeda-Zuñiga, M.D.

Percutaneous needle biopsy of the lung is often preferred over open surgical biopsy because of its high rate of diagnostic accuracy and its low frequency of major complications. It can provide tissue samples for microbiologic, cytologic, and, in some cases, histologic studies, thus potentially identifying with specificity the etiology of pulmonary abnormalities.

In the United States, transthoracic needle aspiration has been accepted and widely used only for the past two decades, despite early reports of the basic technique. Leyden[12] was the first to use percutaneous lung biopsy in the diagnosis of pneumonia. In the first half of this century, suspected infectious processes were biopsied with fine needles and suspected malignant processes with larger needles. Major complications were reported much more commonly in the diagnosis of cancerous lesions when large-bore (3 mm diameter or greater) and cutting-type needles were used.[27] Reports of these complications, which included hemorrhage, tension pneumothorax, and death, dulled enthusiasm for the technique until the 1960s, when Dahlgren and Nordenstrom[4] reported on the use of fluoroscopically guided fine-needle aspiration in the diagnosis of cancer. They achieved a high rate of diagnostic accuracy; additionally, a lower rate of complications was seen compared with the earlier reports with larger needles.

Over the past two decades, improved fluoroscopic equipment and refined needle design have enhanced the technique. For example, with modern image intensification, biopsy of nodules as small as 5 mm in diameter is possible. These technical advances have been accompanied by increased acceptance of cytology as an accurate method of diagnosis.

LESION LOCALIZATION

Three-dimensional localization of the lesion must be accomplished before the biopsy procedure is initiated. This begins with a conventional posteroanterior and lateral radiographic examination of the chest (Fig 2–1,A and B). Plain tomography may be helpful in localizing small lesions, especially if these are not well visualized on the lateral projection, and in detecting multiple lesions (Fig 2–2). With tomography, the depth of the lesion in relation to the skin surface can be estimated. The presence or absence of calcification and cavitation can also be assessed.

Computed tomography is particularly useful in characterizing central and mediastinal lesions. It, as well as nuclear flow studies and angiography, is occasionally required to determine if a more centrally located mass is an aortic aneurysm or other vascular structure.

Fluoroscopic localization prior to the procedure substantiates that a lesion is intrapulmonary and assesses its relationship to blood vessels, pleura, and ribs. Fluoroscopic equipment with good image resolution is essential for biopsy of lesions 2 cm or less in diameter. A biplane or movable C-arm unit is desirable when performing transthoracic biopsy on smaller lesions.

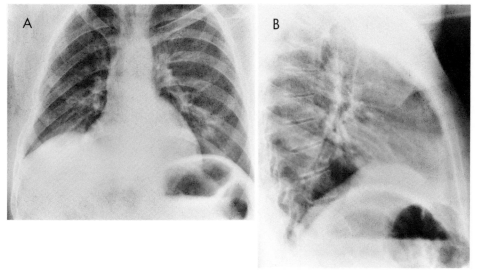

FIG 2–1.
A, chest film, posteroanterior view. Nodular lesion in left base overlies the tip of the fourth left rib. **B,** lateral chest film. The location of the nodule in the left lower lobe is corroborated.

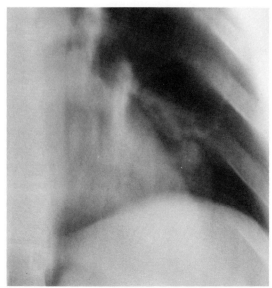

FIG 2–2.
AP tomogram confirms the presence of a
nodule located posteriorly in the left lower
lobe.

TECHNIQUE

Biopsy Needles

Several kinds of biopsy needles suitable for thoracic biopsy are commercially available, including aspiration, cutting, and screw-type needles. Fine-needles are preferred for use in biopsy of intrapulmonary lesions, despite their flexibility, which can make control of needle placement more difficult. Larger needles are better suited for biopsy of pleural-based and some mediastinal lesions.

The 22- and 23-gauge Chiba or Turner[22] needles are frequently used for percutaneous thoracic aspiration biopsy. These can provide microbiologic and cytologic specimens for evaluation. Histologic core specimens can also be obtained with this type of needle; however, use of a cutting-type needle will enhance the likelihood of this occurrence. These include the Greene,[9] Franseen,[1] Sure-cut, and Westcott[25] needles. The even larger 17-gauge Lee[11] and 14-gauge Tru-cut[8] needles can be used in selected mediastinal and pleural-based lesions. The screw-type Rotex biopsy instrument[16] can also be used for thoracic biopsy.

Patient Preparation and General Considerations

Patient preparation for percutaneous transthoracic biopsy is minimal. Sedation is not necessary, but premedication may be warranted in some circumstances. The patient must be able to control his or her breathing, however, making oversedation undesirable. A short period of fasting, approximately eight hours, is often ordered but not essential.

Preliminary laboratory work should include complete blood cell (CBC) and platelet counts and prothrombin and partial thromboplastin times. Appropriate measures to correct hematologic abnormalities should be undertaken before the procedure has begun. Prior to positioning the patient, 10 ml of blood can be drawn and set aside in a syringe to clot. It can then be injected through the needle as it is retracted, in an attempt to seal the needle tract.[14]

The shortest, most direct approach to the lesion is determined by review of previous radiologic studies. Based on this, the patient is positioned prone or supine. If the patient is prone, the hands should be placed under the forehead; if the patient is supine, the hands should be placed behind the head. These positions will facilitate visualization of the lesion on the lateral fluoroscopic view and will help maintain a fixed relationship between the puncture site on the skin and the underlying lesion.

The puncture site is localized fluoroscopically and marked. If possible, to decrease the risk of pneumothorax, only one pulmonary lobe should be entered and no fissures crossed. The puncture site should be chosen as to avoid the intercostal neurovascular bundles located near the inferior aspect of the rib. If biplane fluoroscopy is used, the lesion should be localized in the lateral view as well. Choice of the puncture site should accommodate the following considerations: (1) biopsy of a presumed large tumor should be made from the periphery of the lesion, as the center is often composed of necrotic tissue and debris; and (2) biopsy of a suspected inflammatory lesion should be performed with a more central puncture.

The skin is cleaned with a sterile solution and sterile drapes are placed around the intended puncture site. Local anesthesia is administered, infiltrating the skin, subcutaneous tissue, and intercostal muscle while attempting to not penetrate the parietal pleura. A small dermatomy is made with a scalpel blade.

Needle placements are made during suspended quiet respiration. This can be done in small increments with frequent intermittent fluoroscopic checks and appropriate angular corrections. Alternatively, continuous fluoroscopic control can be used, holding the needle with a forceps. If possible, the needle should be advanced along the fluoroscopic beam, so that the hub and tip are superimposed on the image (Fig 2–3,A). The presence of ribs, scapula, and diaphragm may sometimes preclude this technique and necessitate a slightly angulated needle path. Often a change in tissue consistency is encountered as the needle enters the lesion. The accurate position of the needle tip can be confirmed by biplane or angled fluoroscopy (Fig 2–3,B). Fluoroscopic assessment of the relative movement of the needle tip and the lesion with respiration or even a lateral film may be necessary to confirm positioning of the needle tip within the target lesion.

Wet or dry aspiration biopsy tissue can be performed. With a wet aspiration, a small amount of sterile nonbacteriostatic saline is placed in the syringe.

Immediately on completion of the procedure, a chest film should be taken to assess the possibility of complicating pneumothorax. A delayed film, taken four to six hours later, is also recommended.

Specific Techniques

A simple aspiration biopsy can be performed with a Chiba or Turner needle. Traditionally, this is done with a dry syringe and it obtains material for cytologic and bacteriologic examinations. Rotating the Turner needle during aspi-

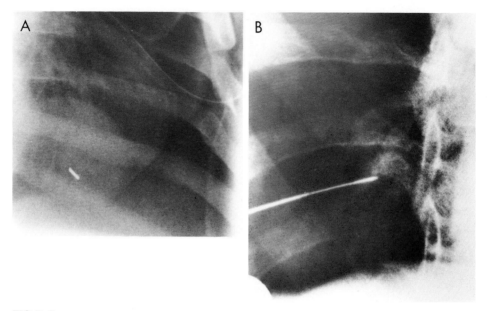

FIG 2–3.
AP film taken during needle insertion shows the almost perpendicular path of the needle. **B,** lateral film during needle advancement shows tip of the needle within the nodule.

ration seems to increase the likelihood of obtaining a tissue core.[13] The needle and stylet are positioned under fluoroscopic control, with the tip situated at the periphery of the target lesion. The needle path should be corrected before the visceral pleura is entered, if possible. While the patient holds his breath, the stylet is removed and a 6- or 12-ml syringe is attached to the needle hub with polyethylene connector tubing. Constant negative pressure is applied as the needle is advanced the short distance into the target lesion and as it is withdrawn.

With a cutting needle, cutting and coring of a histologic specimen are often accompanied by a rotary movement of the needle as it is advanced into the lesion, helping to free tissue from the lesion as it is cut. Suction is maintained as the needle is advanced into the lesion and as it is withdrawn. With cutting needles, such as the Tru-cut, that have a biopsy notch on an inner obturator, the specimen is obtained by advancing the obturator from the cannula into the lesion. The tissue is then cut by advancing the outer cannula. The entire assembly is then withdrawn.

Biopsy with the Rotex instrument is accomplished differently.[16] The assembled instrument is brought to the edge of the lesion. The inner screw needle is advanced until the screw tip has passed into the lesion. The outer cannula is advanced over the screw tip, cutting the tissue core. The cannula and screw are withdrawn together.

These basic biopsy techniques can be adapted to the special circumstances of percutaneous thoracic biopsy. Tandem, coaxial[7] and modified[23] coaxial methods of needle localization can all be used in this setting, using fluoroscopic guidance for needle positioning. The coaxial (Fig 2–4) and modified coaxial

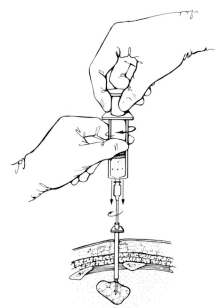

FIG 2–4.
A 19-gauge spinal needle is placed with its tip next to the lesion. A Chiba needle is introduced through the spinal needle for multiple aspirations.

methods allow several passes of the fine biopsy needle into the lesion to be made with only a single penetration of the visceral pleura with a larger introducing needle.

RESULTS

Percutaneous lung biopsy is most useful in the diagnosis of malignancy. A retrospective analysis of the literature cites a sensitivity or true-positive rate of 83% and a specificity or true-negative rate of 98% in the diagnosis of malignancy in 1,826 patients who underwent aspiration biopsy.[18] In review of 215 patients who underwent screw-needle biopsy, sensitivity was 89% and specificity was 98%.[18] Greene[7] cited a positive diagnosis of greater than 95% in lung cancers with a tissue-coring coaxial aspiration technique.

These statistics indicate a false-negative rate of approximately 5% to 10%. The most common cause of a false-negative result is probably inaccurate needle placement. Consequently, needle position should be documented during the procedure with radiographs taken of both the anteroposterior or posteroanterior and lateral projections, if possible. Other causes of false-negative results include aspiration of necrotic material within the tumor or of inflammatory reactions surrounding the neoplasm. Multiple aspirations appear to increase the diagnostic accuracy by minimizing these factors.[28] False-positive diagnosis of malignancy is very rare,[21] and is reported at 0.2% in a Massachusetts General Hospital series.[7]

Percutaneous lung biopsy is much less valuable in identifying the specific etiology of benign neoplasms or noninfectious inflammatory lesions. Greene[7] noted that a specific diagnosis can be made in only 10% of the benign lesions with the dry aspiration cytologic method and in 40% with the wet aspiration histologic tissue-core technique.

Percutaneous lung biopsy has, however, been of considerable benefit in the diagnosis of infectious pulmonary disease, especially in high-risk and immunocompromised hosts.[2, 3, 19] Accuracy of the diagnosis in these patients depends not only on adequate specimen aspiration, but also on appropriate culture and staining techniques. Anaerobic culture material must be transported in a special medium or in a capped, air-free syringe. Other culture media may be necessary for viral agents. Cooperation with the pathologist and infectious disease specialist may be necessary to provide material for all of the desired diagnostic tests.

COMPLICATIONS

The most common complications of percutaneous lung biopsy are pneumothorax and hemorrhage. The frequency of detectable pneumothorax after this procedure ranges from 14% to 57%.[5, 6, 10, 15] Greene[7] stated that the prevalence of pneumothorax with the coaxial technique is between 10% and 15%, with only approximately 5% of patients requiring aspiration and/or chest tube placement for large or symptomatic pneumothoraces. Pneumothorax occurring during the course of the procedure can make aspiration of the target lesion difficult. The chest should be fluoroscopically examined immediately after the procedure to detect shift of the midline structures or even more direct evidence of a pneumothorax. An immediate upright anteroposterior or posteroanterior chest film is obtained, as is another film four to six hours after the biopsy, as small leaks may have a delayed presentation as pneumothorax. Of course, any change in the patient's symptoms that would suggest pneumothorax warrants prompt radiographic and clinical evaluation.

Attention to technical details can minimize the risk of pneumothorax after percutaneous lung biopsy. A single pass through the visceral pleura is optimal. If a coaxial technique is used, the introducing needle, once in position, should remain deep to the visceral pleura. A small amount of sterile nonbacteriostatic saline can be placed on the hub of the introducing needle during the procedure and an autologous blood clot can be injected into the needle on withdrawal as precautionary measures against development of pneumothorax.

Hemorrhage after percutaneous lung biopsy can take the form of hemoptysis or local parenchymal hemorrhage. The frequency of hemoptysis has been variably reported as 3% to 10%; the condition is usually self-limited and not severe.[5, 6, 10, 15] Local parenchymal hemorrhage need not be accompanied by hemoptysis, but is often asymptomatic and detected only by radiographic examination. It usually resolves spontaneously in 48 to 72 hours. Performing the procedure in patients with normal or corrected bleeding values will minimize the risk of both of these complications.

Other nonfatal complications are much less common and include air embolism[24] and tumor implantation along the needle tract.[26] Both seem to be more frequent with the use of large-caliber needles. Other complications are rare. Subcutaneous and mediastinal emphysema have been reported, as have chest wall hematomas and pleural infections.[20]

Fatal complications of percutaneous lung biopsy are uncommon and, as with nonfatal complications, have been reported with greatest frequency with the use of large-caliber needles. The risk of death with fine-needle aspiration has been estimated to be less than 0.02%.[7] The causes of reported deaths have been related to air embolism and pulmonary hemorrhage.[17, 24]

CONTRAINDICATIONS

Contraindications to percutaneous needle biopsy of the lung are generally relative and are related in large part to the major risks of the procedure, pneumothorax and bleeding. Pneumothorax is poorly tolerated in patients with severe pulmonary disease. This is especially true for those with significant airway obstruction (less than 50% predicted flow rates) and hypoxemia (PaO_2 less than 60 mm Hg). The need for the procedure must be carefully weighed against the potential risks in each individual case. Preparations for expeditious treatment with a thoracotomy tube should be made prior to the initiation of the biopsy in these patients.

The potential risk of pneumothorax is somewhat increased if bullous disease is present in the region of the target lesion. This represents only a relative contraindication to needle biopsy, as pneumothorax can be readily controlled with the placement of a thoracotomy tube.

Bleeding from a transthoracic needle biopsy can be serious. In light of this risk, any tendency for bleeding should be identified by preliminary laboratory work. Hematologic consultation may be necessary for abnormalities not easily corrected. For patients receiving therapeutic anticoagulation, biopsy can be performed on the day that heparin therapy is stopped, and, if necessary, reversed with protamine sulfate.

Patients with pulmonary arterial hypertension are at increased risk for bleeding from needle biopsy. Again the need for the procedure must be determined on an individual basis in these patients. Pulmonary venous hypertension also increases the risk of bleeding; however, it does not preclude the procedure unless concomitant pulmonary edema is present.

A few special circumstances may represent contraindications to the procedure. An uncooperative patient or one with an uncontrollable cough may not be a suitable candidate. Increased risk of air embolism is seen in patients on positive-pressure respirators and this should be taken into account when the procedure is considered in these patients. Percutaneous aspiration biopsy should be avoided in patients with suspected echinococcal cysts, as anaphylaxis may occur and cyst rupture may lead to the development of daughter cysts.

CONCLUSION

Percutaneous thoracic aspiration is a relatively safe procedure now performed regularly in many institutions. Accurate localization is essential to an accurate procedure and can be accomplished frequently with fluoroscopy. Both fine- and larger gauge needles can be used for biopsy, with fine-needles suitable for parenchymal, pleural, hilar, and mediastinal lesions, and larger gauge needles suitable only for some pleural and mediastinal lesions.

REFERENCES

1. Ballard GL, Boyd WR: A specially designed cutting aspiration needle for lung biopsy. *AJR* 1978; 130:899–903.
2. Bandt PD, Blank N, Castellino RA: Needle diagnosis of pneumonitis. Value in high-risk patients. *JAMA* 1972; 220:1578–1580.
3. Castellino RA, Blank N: Etiologic diagnosis of focal pulmonary infection in immunocompromised patients by fluoroscopically guided percutaneous needle aspiration. *Radiology* 1979; 132:562–567.
4. Dahlgren S, Nordenstrom B: *Transthoracic Needle Biopsy.* Chicago, Year Book Medical Publishers Inc, 1966.
5. Fontana RS, et al: Transthoracic needle aspiration of discrete pulmonary lesions: Experience in 100 cases. *Med Clin North Am* 1977; 54:961–971.
6. Francis D: Aspiration biopsies from diagnostically difficult pulmonary lesions: Experience in 100 cases. *Med Clin North Am* 1970; 54:961–971.
7. Greene RF: Transthoracic needle aspiration biopsy, in Athanasoulis CA, et al (eds): *Interventional Radiology.* Philadelphia, WB Saunders Co, 1982, pp. 587–634.
8. Haaga JR, et al: Clinical comparison of small and large caliber cutting needles for biopsy. *Radiology* 1983; 146:665–667.
9. Isler RJ, et al: Tissue core biopsy of abdominal tumors with a 22-gauge cutting needle. *AJR* 1981; 136:725–729.
10. Lalli AF, et al: Aspiration biopsies of chest lesions. *Radiology* 1978; 127:35–40.
11. Lee LH: A new biopsy needle and its clinical use. *AJR* 1974; 121:854–859.
12. Leyden E: Über infektiose pneumonie. *Dtsch Med Wochenschr* 1883; 9:52–54.
13. Lieberman RP, Hafez JR, Crummy AB: Histology from aspiration biopsy: Turner needle experience. *AJR* 1982; 138:561–564.
14. McCartney R, et al: A technique for prevention of pneumothorax in pulmonary aspiration biopsy. *AJR* 1974; 120:872–875.
15. Meyer JE, et al: Percutaneous aspiration biopsy of nodular lung lesions. *J Thorac Cardiovasc Surg* 1977; 73:787–791.
16. Nordenstrom B: New instrument for biopsy. *Radiology* 1975; 117:474–475.
17. Pearce JG, Patt NL: Fatal pulmonary hemorrhage after percutaneous aspiration lung biopsy. *Am Rev Respir Dis* 1974; 110:346–349.
18. Poe RH, Tobin RE: Sensitivity and specificity of needle biopsy in lung malignancy. *Am Rev Respir Dis* 1980; 122:725–729.
19. Ramsey PG, et al: The renal transplant patient with fever and pulmonary infiltrates: Etiology, clinical manifestations, and management. *Medicine* 1980; 59:206–222.
20. Sinner WN: Complications of percutaneous transthoracic needle aspiration biopsy. *Acta Radiol (Diagn) (Stockh)* 1976; 17:813–828.
21. Taft PD, Szyfelbein WM, Greene RF: Variability in pulmonary cytologic diagnosis. *Am J Clin Pathol* 1980; 73:36–40.
22. Turner AF, Sargent EN: Percutaneous pulmonary needle biopsy. *AJR* 1968; 104:846–850.
23. vanSonnenberg E, et al: Percutaneous biopsy of difficult mediastinal, hilar and

pulmonary lesions by computed tomographic guidance and a modified coaxial technique. *Radiology* 1983; 148:300–302.

24. Westcott JL: Air embolism complicating percutaneous needle biopsy of the lung. *Chest* 1973; 63:108–110.

25. Westcott JL: Direct percutaneous needle aspiration of localized pulmonary lesions: Results in 432 patients. *Radiology* 1980; 137:31–35.

26. Wolinsky H, Lischner MW: Needle track implantation of tumor after percutaneous lung biopsy. *Ann Intern Med* 1969; 71:359–362.

27. Woolf CR: Applications of aspiration lung biopsy with a review of the literature. *Dis Chest* 1954; 25:286–300.

28. Zornoza J: Lung and pleura, in Zornoza J (ed): *Percutaneous Needle Biopsy.* Baltimore, Williams and Wilkins Co, 1981, pp. 52–77.

3

Percutaneous Aspiration of Thoracic Fluid Collections and Masses With Ultrasound Guidance

Janis G. Letourneau, M.D.
Morteza K. Elyaderani, M.D.

During ultrasonography of the chest, echoes are generated from the skin, intercostal muscles, and parietal pleura. At a depth of approximately 3.5 cm, the ultrasonic waves are reflected from the air-tissue interface at the surface of the lung.[6,12] Although lesions deep within the lung are not well visualized by ultrasound (US), the procedure is effective in demonstrating the pleura, the pleural space, and the immediate subpleural region of the lung. In comparison to the normal air-tissue interface, there is generally a decrease in the magnitude of reflection from diseased surfaces.[14]

Ultrasonography is superior to radiographic techniques for detecting small, loculated collections of pleural fluid and for differentiating these from pleural thickening.[1,8] Ultrasonography also may be useful in differentiating effusions, which may be tapped or drained, from neoplastic lesions.[7]

ULTRASONOGRAPHY OF NORMALLY AERATED LUNG

The marked difference in the acoustic impedances of the soft tissues of the chest wall and of aerated lung results in complete reflection of the sound beam at their interface.[13] It is not possible to demonstrate a mass or fluid collection

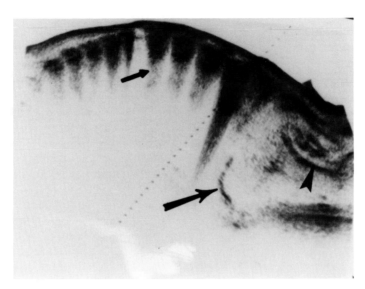

FIG 3–1.
Prone longitudinal sonogram shows the normal posterior aspect of right hemithorax. The diaphragm *(large arrow)*, reverberation *(small arrow)*, and kidney *(arrowhead)* are shown.

in the lung if air intervenes between the lesion and the chest wall. A normal sonogram of the lung demonstrates skin, subcutaneous fat, intercostal muscles, and the parietal layer of the pleura. Aerated lung totally reflects the sound beam, but triangular reverberation echoes are seen. Rib interference is critical because the acoustic window for imaging the lung is small. The area beneath the ribs is free of echoes because of absorption, reflection, and scattering of the sound beam (Fig 3–1).

PLEURAL EFFUSION

Pleural effusion can be diagnosed with confidence in most patients by a chest radiograph, but subpulmonary effusion is sometimes difficult to detect by this method. It is generally accepted that 300 to 500 ml of free fluid must be present in the pleural cavity to be seen on a posteroanterior upright chest film. Decubitus views may demonstrate a pleural fluid volume of approximately 100 ml. The value of US in detecting small pleural effusions is well established. Gryminski et al.[8] reported that it is useful in accurately localizing even very small collections of fluid, although the minimum amount of fluid that can be detected has not yet been determined. Therefore, when the chest radiograph is indeterminate and the presence or absence of fluid is clinically significant, US is a valuable imaging modality.

Ultrasonographic Method of Detecting Pleural Effusion

Evaluation of the patient for nonloculated pleural effusion requires examination with the patient in a sitting position. This allows free fluid to flow into the most dependent, posterior portion of the pleural space. The examiner attempts to localize the diaphragm and the posterior costophrenic angles. This is most easily accomplished with a real-time scanner. The fluid appears as echo-free space just above the diaphragm in the posterior costophrenic angle (Fig 3–2,A). A large amount of pleural effusion also can be demonstrated with the patient in the lateral decubitus position, using the liver (or spleen) as the acoustic window (Fig 3–2,B and C).

Loculated pleural effusions, such as hematoma (Fig 3–3) or empyema (Fig 3–4), appear as sharply demarcated, echo-free spaces protruding into the hemithorax and compressing contiguous lung. Low-level echoes may be detected in these fluid collections. The presence of an echo-free space does not prove that the fluid is in the pleural cavity, since an intraparenchymal fluid collection such as a lung abscess, cyst, or tumor (Fig 3–5) cannot be differentiated easily from a loculated pleural effusion. Acoustic enhancement beyond the posterior wall of a fluid collection is not seen in the chest, since the interface is air containing and will be strongly echogenic. Use of a higher frequency, focused transducer or even a waterbath over the chest to bring the lesion into the focal zone of the transducer may be helpful.

Aspiration of Pleural Effusion Under Guidance of Ultrasound

Thoracentesis under the guidance of US is simple and accurate. It decreases complications such as pneumothorax and inadvertent puncture of the aerated

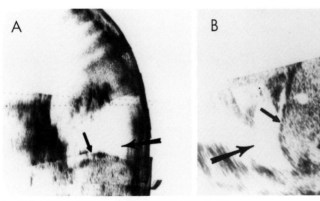

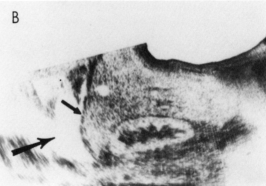

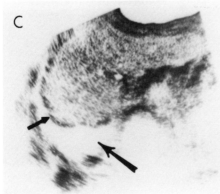

FIG 3–2.
A, longitudinal sonogram of the posterior aspect of the right hemithorax with the patient sitting shows a pleural effusion *(large arrow)* and the diaphragm *(small arrow)*. **B,** decubitus longitudinal sonogram of the right upper quadrant shows the diaphragm *(small arrow)* and pleural effusion *(large arrow)*. **C,** decubitus transverse sonogram of right upper quadrant shows pleural effusion *(large arrow)* and the diaphragm *(small arrow)*.

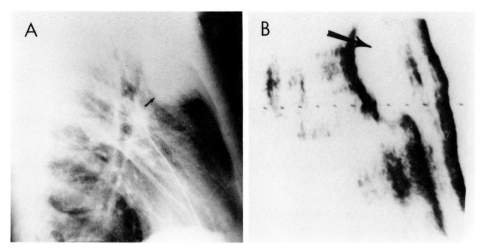

FIG 3–3.
A, lateral chest view shows a soft-tissue mass in retrosternal region *(small arrow).* **B,** anterior longitudinal sonogram of corresponding retrosternal mass, which is echo free *(large arrow).* Fine-needle aspiration demonstrated a hematoma.

lung, liver, spleen, and kidney because of more precise needle placement. Aspiration of pleural fluid can be performed as either a diagnostic or therapeutic procedure.

The nature of the fluid cannot be solely determined by its sonographic features. In fact, some authors have found it difficult to predict which pleural

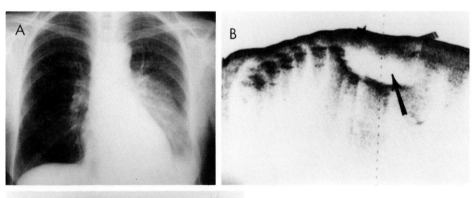

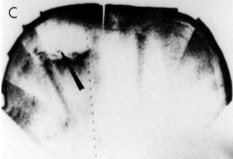

FIG 3–4.
A, posteroanterior chest film shows a soft-tissue density on the left lung. **B,** prone longitudinal sonogram shows that the corresponding soft-tissue mass is a fluid collection *(large arrow).* **C,** prone transverse sonogram of the same patient with empyema. Note low-level echoes in the dependent portion of the abscess cavity *(large arrow).*

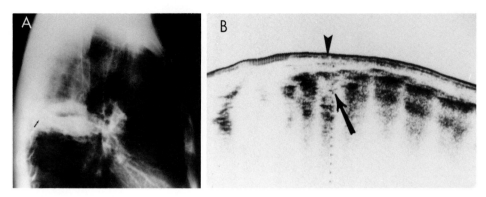

FIG 3–5.
A, lateral chest roentgenogram demonstrates a posterior soft-tissue mass with air-fluid level. There is a narrow area of contiguity to the chest wall *(short arrow).* **B,** prone longitudinal sonogram shows a poorly defined mass *(large arrow).* Aspiration confirmed malignancy with central necrosis. *Arrowhead* points to site of needle puncture.

collections can be drained, since echo-free lesions may not yield fluid, while complex appearing lesions may.[2,10]

The effusion is localized with the available equipment, either linear-array or sector real-time or static B-mode scanner. Complementary A-mode scanning is helpful in determining the angle of approach and is sometimes used in our patients.

The site of the puncture should be over the most dependent portion of the fluid for either diagnostic or therapeutic thoracentesis. The point of entry should be at the upper margin of the nearest rib to avoid damage to intercostal neurovascular bundles. The puncture site is marked on the skin and the area is sterilized. The tissues are anesthetized down to the parietal pleura. After administration of local anesthesia, a small caliber needle is inserted to the predetermined depth and angle while the patient holds his breath. The stylet of the needle is removed, and the needle hub is connected to a syringe and plastic tubing for aspiration. The patient can breathe normally after insertion of the needle. Aspiration of only a small amount of fluid is required for a diagnostic thoracentesis. The aspirate is sent for Gram stain, culture and sensitivity, and cytopathologic examination.

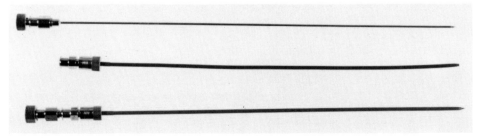

FIG 3–6.
Translumbar aortography set can be used to drain thoracic fluid collections.

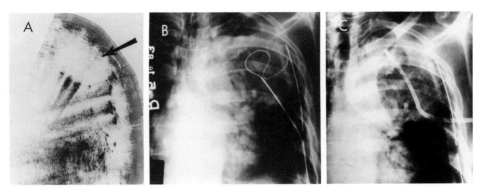

FIG 3–7.
A, longitudinal sonogram demonstrates a large thoracic fluid collection *(large arrow).* **B,** prone film of left upper lung field shows a guidewire situated in the abscess cavity. **C,** posteroanterior chest view shows a 14-F catheter, with multiple side holes, in the abscess cavity.

More complete evacuation of the pleural space is required for a therapeutic procedure. If desired, a catheter can be placed in the pleural space for drainage using standard Seldinger technique following diagnostic aspiration. An 18-gauge needle (Fig 3–6) is inserted parallel to the fine-aspiration needle in tandem fashion. The stylet of the needle is removed and aspiration of a small amount of fluid is performed to verify the location of the needle tip in the fluid collection. A guidewire is inserted and the needle is removed (Fig 3–7A, B, and C). The tract is dilated to the size of the drainage catheter (Fig 3–8). An 8- to 12- French (F) catheter with a straight (Fig 3–9) or pigtail end and multiple side holes (Fig 3–10) is advanced over the guidewire into the pleural

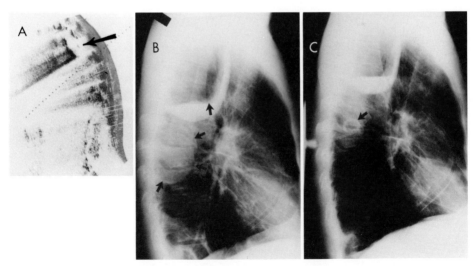

FIG 3–8.
A, longitudinal sonogram demonstrates a posterior fluid collection *(arrow).* **B,** lateral chest film shows a soft-tissue mass *(large arrows)* with a large cavity demonstrating air-fluid level seen superiorly *(upper arrow).* **C,** lateral chest film shows a pigtail catheter draining the empyema cavity.

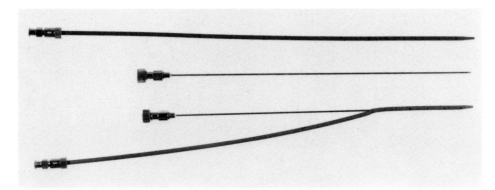

FIG 3–9.
Pneumothorax set that can be used to drain thoracic or fluid collections.

collection and connected to a bag or to regulated suction. Effective evacuation requires that all loculations be drained. The exudative stage of empyema may also be treated in such a fashion; however, a more chronic empyema may not be effectively treated with percutaneous drainage, and a surgical procedure may be required (Fig 3–11). On the other hand, US has been used to guide successful drainage of empyema when conventional thoracostomy tube drainage has failed.[15]

THORACIC MASS

Ultrasonography is a good means of localizing peripheral lung masses and distinguishing small peripheral lung tumors from pleural thickening or fluid loculation. There is no specific echo pattern for different solid masses of the lung or for pleural-based tumors. A consolidation resulting from pneumonia (Fig 3–12), atelectasis, or infarction cannot be distinguished ultrasonographically from a peripheral pulmonary neoplasm or a pleural-based lesion (Fig 3–13). The exact location of a thoracic lesion may even be difficult to assess, a peripheral pulmonary abscess being indistinguishable from an empyema.[11] It may also be difficult or even impossible to distinguish a cystic mass from a solid one. If the mass is surrounded by air-containing lung in the far wall, acoustic enhancement posterior to a fluid collection and strong artifactual echoes from the interface of air and soft tissue cannot be distinguished (Fig 3–14). Because of these considerations, fine-needle aspiration can be of value in the diagnosis of peripheral lung masses.

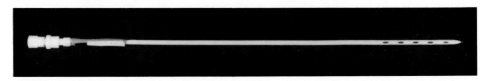

FIG 3–10.
14-F catheter with multiple side holes and trocar stylet.

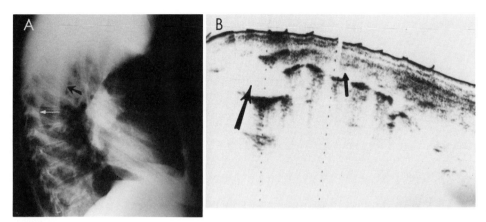

FIG 3–11.
A, lateral chest roentgenogram in a patient with chronic empyema *(large arrow).* **B,** prone longitudinal sonogram shows a large fluid collection *(large arrow)* with extension inferoposteriorly *(small arrow).*

Aspiration Technique

Examinations can be done with a standard diagnostic transducer. Patients are examined in a supine, prone, decubitus, or upright sitting position, depending on the location of the lesion, and in longitudinal and transverse planes usually with a real-time unit.[4,9]

After the mass is localized, the depth and angle for aspiration biopsy are determined (Figs 3–15 and 3–16). Aspiration can be accomplished with a biopsy transducer, although use of such a transducer is not essential; however, precise localization of the lesion is necessary.[6]

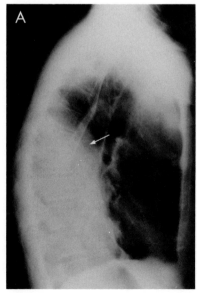

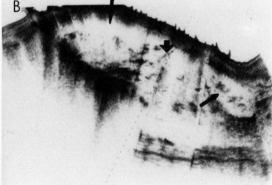

FIG 3–12.
A, lateral chest film shows a soft-tissue density in the posterior aspect of the hemithorax *(small arrow).* **B,** prone longitudinal sonogram demonstrates the mass is primarily solid *(large arrow).* Aspiration biopsy specimen proved the mass was not malignant, but was a chronic nonspecific pneumonia. The diaphragm is noted *(arrowhead),* as is the kidney *(small arrow).*

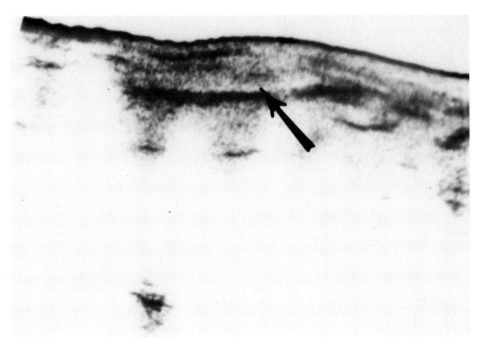

FIG 3–13.
Decubitus sonogram shows metastatic pleural thickening *(arrow)* in a patient with carcinoma of the breast.

RESULTS

Success rates for fine-needle aspiration of lung masses under US guidance have approached 100% with no false-negative results.[6] The most frequent complications of fine-needle aspiration of thoracic lesions are pain (23%), pneumothorax (19%), and hemoptysis (16%).[5] The rate of pneumothorax is even higher (49%) in older patients and in those with cavitating and mediastinal

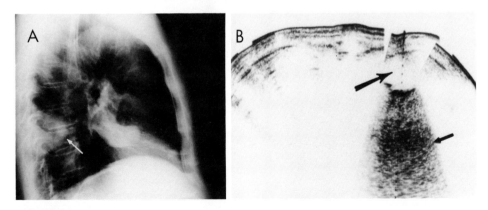

FIG 3–14.
A, lateral chest roentgenogram shows multiple soft-tissue masses in a patient with primary hypernephroma *(arrow)*. **B,** transverse sonogram demonstrates a mass without obvious internal echoes *(large arrow)* and strong false acoustic enhancement *(small arrow)*. Aspiration biopsy by 22-gauge needle confirmed the solid nature of the mass, a metastatic focus of hypernephroma.

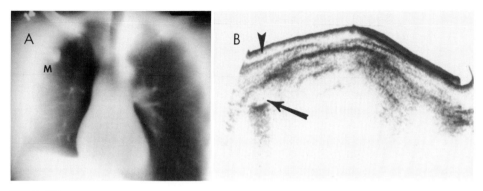

FIG 3–15.
A, anteroposterior tomogram reveals sharply circumscribed nodule in the right upper lung field. (From Elyaderani MK, Gabriele OF: *Southern Med J* 1982; 75:536–539. Reproduced by permission.) M indicates mass. **B,** supine transverse sonogram of the same patient reveals a sharply defined solid mass *(arrow)* measuring 1.5 cm in diameter that proved to be a metastasis from carcinoma of the breast. Needle puncture site is indicated by *arrowhead.*

lesions when a large gauge needle is used, with 5% of these patients requiring thoracostomy tube placement.[3] Malignant seeding of the tract after fine-needle aspiration has been reported.[6]

SUMMARY

Ultrasonography is a useful and relatively safe modality for detecting peripheral intrathoracic lesions and for directing diagnostic or therapeutic aspiration.

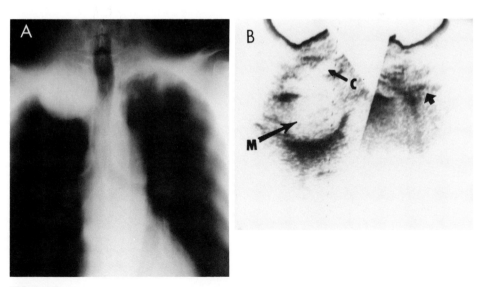

FIG 3–16.
A, anteroposterior lung tomogram shows a soft-tissue mass in right apical region. **B,** supine transverse sonogram reveals it to be a solid mass (M) *(large arrow).* Note the right common carotid artery (C) *(small arrow).* Acoustic shadowing from the trachea *(arrowhead)* is seen in the midline.

REFERENCES

1. Adams FV, Galati V: M-Mode ultrasonic localization of pleural effusion. *JAMA* 1978; 239:1761.
2. Alexander JC Jr, Wolfe WG: Lung abscess and empyema of the thorax. *Surg Clin North Am* 1980; 60:835–849.
3. Berquist TH, et al: Transthoracic needle biopsy. *Mayo Clin Proc* 1980; 55:475–581.
4. Cinti D, Hawkins HB: Aspiration biopsy of peripheral pulmonary masses using real-time sonographic guidance. *AJR* 1984; 142:1115–1116.
5. Ekstrand KE, Blake DD, Dixon RL: Ultrasonography of the chest wall. *J Clin Ultrasound* 1974; 2:117–118.
6. Elyaderani MK, Gabriele OF: Aspiration of thoracic masses and fluid collections under guidance of ultrasonography. *South Med J* 1982; 75:436–439.
7. Forsberg L, Tylen U: Ultrasound examination of lesions in the thorax. *Acta Radiol* 1980; 21:375–378.
8. Gryminski J, Krakowka P, Lypacewicz G: The diagnosis of pleural effusion by ultrasonic and radiologic techniques. *Chest* 1976; 70:33–37.
9. Ikezoe J, et al: Sonographically guided needle biopsy for diagnosis of thoracic lesions. *AJR* 1984; 143:229–234.
10. Laing FC, Filly RA: Problems in the application of ultrasonography in the evaluation of pleural opacities. *Radiology* 1978; 126:211–214.
11. Landay MJ, Conrad MR: Lung abscess mimicking empyema on ultrasonography. *AJR* 1979; 133:731–734.
12. Majan J: The usefulness of needle biopsy in chest lesions of different sizes and locations. *Radiology* 1978; 134:13–15.
13. Sagar KB, et al: Characterization of normal and abnormal pulmonary surface by reflected ultrasound. *Chest* 1978; 74:29–33.
14. Sandweiss DA: Empyema or abscess? Is ultrasound a diagnostic aid? *Chest* 1979; 75:297–298.
15. vanSonnenberg E, et al: CT- and ultrasound-guided catheter drainage of empyemas after chest-tube failure. *Radiology* 1984; 151:349–353.

Percutaneous Aspiration and Drainage of Thoracic Masses With Computed Tomographic Guidance

Janis G. Letourneau, M.D.

Fluoroscopic guidance is the time-honored means of localization for transthoracic biopsy or drainage. Ultrasound (US) localization of peripheral thoracic lesions is also valuable. Some lesions, however, are not well seen fluoroscopically or sonographically because of their position, size, or density and are better imaged with computed tomography (CT) for biopsy localization. This is especially true for more central, hilar, and mediastinal lesions and for more ill-defined small, peripheral parenchymal lesions. Thoracic drainage can also be accomplished with CT guidance and doing so presents its own specific set of technical advantages, as well as limitations.

ASPIRATION BIOPSY OF SOLID OR COMPLEX THORACIC MASSES

As with all percutaneous biopsy procedures, accurate localization of the lesion is essential for a safe and accurate transthoracic needle aspiration. Small, and sometimes even large, parenchymal lesions that may not be seen well fluoroscopically may be easily visualized with CT (Fig 4–1,A and B). Detectability on plain radiographs (Fig 4–1,C and D) will often be predictive of visibility under

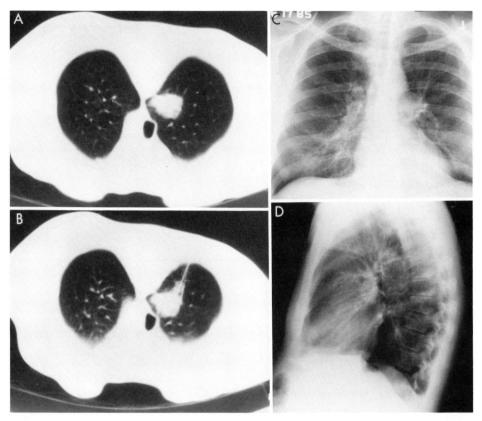

FIG 4–1.
A, CT of a right upper lobe lung mass with the patient in a prone position. **B,** biopsy of the same lung mass with a fine needle. **C,** posteroanterior chest demonstrating the relatively poor visualization of the right upper lobe mass because of overlying bony structures. **D,** mass was also not well seen on the lateral chest view.

fluoroscopy. Perihilar, hilar, and mediastinal lesions may not be clearly separable from vascular structures fluoroscopically, and therefore may be more safely biopsied with CT guidance.[4] Computed tomography can be used in conjunction with fluoroscopy for biopsy of central thoracic lesions.[2] Enhancement of the hilar and mediastinal vascular structures with intravenous (IV) contrast administration may also be of value in this setting (Fig 4–2). Pleural-based masses or pleural or subpleural fluid collections can also be localized with CT if necessary.[5] The major disadvantage of CT localization for transthoracic biopsy is its inability to provide for continuous monitoring of needle position during placement.

Localization of the lesion in the transaxial plane is first accomplished. Slight modification in the intended puncture site may need to be made to allow the puncture to pass on the superior aspect of the rib, thereby avoiding the intercostal neurovascular structures. A needle course directly perpendicular to the body surface may not be feasible because of the location of hilar and mediastinal structures. Necessary angulation of the needle path and the distance from

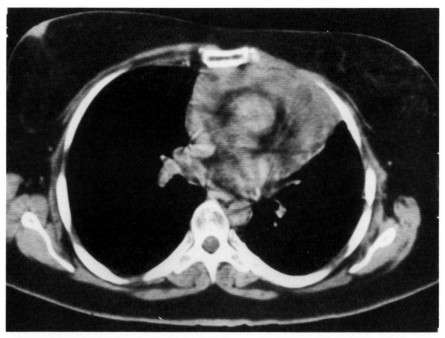

FIG 4–2.
Intravenous contrast was given before biopsy of this large mediastinal mass to verify the location of the aorta and main pulmonary artery.

the skin to the target lesion can be calculated by the CT scanner (Fig 4–3). The patient should be scanned in the position that will allow the shortest intrathoracic needle course that avoids vital structures. This could be a supine, prone, oblique, or decubitus position in the CT scanner gantry. Flexing of the arms above the head in the supine and prone positions moves the scapulae away from the lung fields and facilitates needle placement. Insertion of the needle should be done with the patient in suspended quiet respiration. Respiration can be resumed while the needle position is verified by repeat scanning.

A lower complication rate with fine-needle transthoracic biopsy as compared with larger gauge needle aspiration is clearly established in the literature.[3] Maximal use of fine needles for initial localization is definitely indicated with CT-guided thoracic biopsies, as the needle tip position can only be verified by delayed repeat scans. Consequently, initial placement and redirection should be accomplished with a fine needle in most cases. (Exceptions might include large masses in the mediastinum or in the pleural space or adjacent subpleural locations.) The coaxial technique can be used with the larger outer needle passed in tandem along the fine needle used for initial localization. A modified coaxial technique described by vanSonnenberg et al.[4] also permits multiple biopsy passes without multiple punctures with a larger gauge needle. As initially described, it entailed cutting the hub of the fine localizing needle (22 or 23 gauge) and inserting a larger needle (19 gauge) over the shaft of the fine needle in a coaxial fashion. This allows multiple biopsies to be taken through the

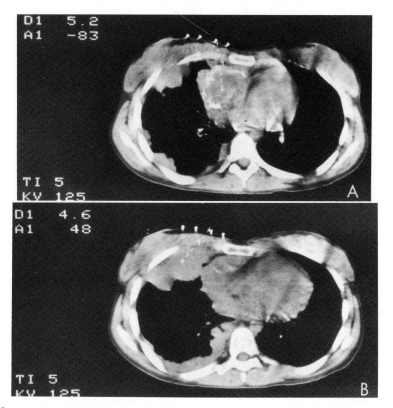

FIG 4–3.
A, distance and angulation measurements obtained from the CT scanner in a young woman with a mediastinal mass. **B,** distance and angulation measurements obtained from the CT scanner in the same patient with subpleural or pleural-based masses. The distance is measured from the skin surface to the lesion. The angulation measurement relates to a horizontal plane, parallel to the CT tabletop.

larger needle. A needle system specifically designed for this modified coaxial technique is now available commercially (Cook Inc.)[6] (Fig 4–4). Both of these methods help avoid inadvertent placement of a larger needle in an inaccurate or undesirable location. All biopsy passes with a fine needle should be made with the patient in suspended respiration.

Some large mediastinal and pleural lesions may be safely biopsied with larger and even cutting-type needles. The absence of intervening lung along the needle path permits the use of this type of needle (Fig 4–5). If the mass is very large and distant from major vascular or airway structures, primary localization can be made and confirmed with the biopsy needle. If this is not the case, a large biopsy needle can be placed in tandem along a fine localizing needle.

Results of CT-guided transthoracic needle aspiration must be viewed in the context of patient selection for this type of procedure. Computed tomography will probably not be the standard method of localization for transthoracic aspiration biopsy, but will be the method of guidance when other imaging modalities fail. Fink et al.[1] reported an overall accuracy of 88% with a sensitivity of 84%. These results were accompanied by a relatively high incidence of pneumothorax (61%), with 11% of the patients requiring thoracostomy tube drainage. This rate of pneumothorax was attributed to the length of time the needle was in place for the procedure, 15 to 20 minutes. An accuracy of 80% was reported with a modified coaxial technique and this was associated with a 10% incidence of pneumothorax.[4]

DRAINAGE OF THORACIC FLUID COLLECTIONS

Computed tomography can be used to localize intrathoracic fluid collections for diagnostic aspiration or for therapeutic aspiration and catheter drainage. The fluid collections suited for this type of procedure will most commonly be

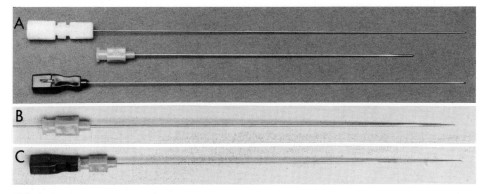

FIG 4–4.
A, the three components of the vanSonnenberg modified coaxial needle biopsy set (Cook, Inc.). The fine-needle at the top has a detachable hub and a diamond tip. The larger needle in the middle is passed over the fine-needle for localization. A Chiba needle, pictured below, is used for biopsy. **B,** the larger needle has been passed over the fine localizing needle once the detachable hub has been removed. **C,** Chiba needle is passed through the larger 19-gauge needle for biopsy.

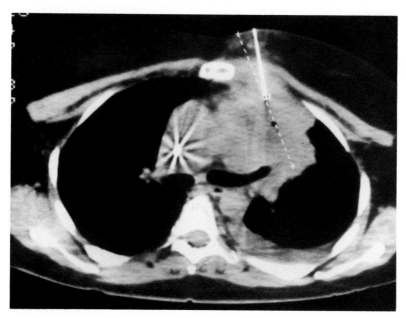

FIG 4–5.
Large anterior mediastinal mass was biopsied directly with a 14-gauge Tru-cut needle following CT localization.

peripheral in location, pleural, or subpleural; however, parenchymal abscesses may also be drained percutaneously with CT guidance. Small, freely dependent pleural effusions are not well suited to aspiration with CT localization because they collect in a location that is inaccessible while the patient is in the CT scanner gantry. Guidance by CT can be used to facilitate percutaneous drainage as a primary therapeutic intervention or it can be used to define the location of fluid following failure of thoracostomy tube drainage.[5]

Localization of the fluid in the transaxial plane is first performed with the patient in a position that allows the lesion to be accessible to a needle or catheter. This may be a supine, prone, oblique, or decubitus position. If catheter drainage is anticipated, posterior or posterolateral puncture site will facilitate drainage in a bedridden patient. Placement of a grid[7] or other marker on the skin precisely localizes the puncture site on repeat scans. Imaging for localization and needle and catheter placement should be performed with the patient in suspended quiet respiration.

Simple aspiration of the fluid can be accomplished with a fine needle (Fig 4–6). Typically, a 22-gauge needle is sufficient, although a 20-gauge needle may be needed if viscous fluid is encountered.[5] Therapeutic aspiration can be attempted with the biopsy needle, if desired. For catheter drainage either standard Seldinger or trocar techniques can be used following localization with a fine needle.[5] Fluoroscopic guidance may be valuable once guidewire, dilator, and catheter manipulations begin. A variety of catheter types and sizes may be used for this procedure, with catheters 8-12 French (F) having some form of terminal curve being used most frequently in a series of percutaneously drained empyemas.[5] These authors also contend that irrigation of thoracic ab-

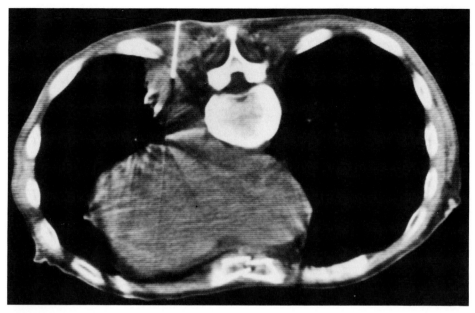

FIG 4–6.
Fine-needle aspiration of a loculated posteriorly situated pleural hematoma noted following cardiac transplantation.

scesses is required less frequently and with less volume than with abdominal abscesses and that Dionosil (Glaxo, Inc.) should be used as the contrast agent for sinograms, because of the possibility of communication of the abscess cavity with the bronchial tree.

Results from the Massachusetts General Hospital series were encouraging, with 100% of patients with empyema drained successfully percutaneously with CT guidance. The empyema cavity in nine of these ten patients also closed. No bleeding or hemothorax occurred in this group of patients.[5]

CONCLUSION

Computed tomographic localization for diagnostic or therapeutic percutaneous procedures in the chest is becoming more widely used. Its major disadvantage is that it does not allow continuous monitoring of the needle or catheter position. It does, however, result in the acquisition of precise anatomic information regarding the relationship of pathological lesions to normal and often vital structures.

REFERENCES

1. Fink I, Gamsu G, Harber LP: CT-guided aspiration biopsy of the thorax. *J Comput Assist Tomogr* 1982; 6:958–962.
2. Gobein RP, Skucas J, Paris BS: CT-assisted fluoroscopically guided aspiration biopsy of central hilar and mediastinal masses. *Radiology* 1981; 141:443–447.

3. Grunze H: A critical review and evaluation of cytodiagnosis in chest diseases. *Acta Cytologica* 1960; 4:175–198.

4. vanSonnenberg E, et al: Percutaneous biopsy of difficult mediastinal, hilar and pulmonary lesions by computed tomographic guidance and a modified coaxial technique. *Radiology* 1983; 148:300–302.

5. vanSonnenberg E, et al: CT- and ultrasound-guided catheter drainage of empyemas after chest-tube failure. *Radiology* 1984; 151:349–353.

6. vanSonnenberg E, et al: Removal hub needle system for coaxial biopsy of small and difficult lesions. *Radiology* 1984; 152:226.

7. Wittenberg J, et al: Percutaneous core biopsy of abdominal tumors using 22-gauge needles: Further observations. *AJR* 1982; 139:75–80.

5

Fluoroscopy-Guided Transabdominal Biopsy of Retroperitoneal Masses

Janis G. Letourneau, M.D.
Yukiyoshi Kimura, M.D.
Wilfrido R. Castañeda-Zuñiga, M.D.

Fine-needle aspiration biopsy of retroperitoneal masses is associated with a high rate of diagnostic accuracy and a low rate of significant complications. As with percutaneous needle biopsy of the lung, this technique is most useful in identifying malignant lesions. Its application can often preclude diagnostic surgery and aid in the planning of therapeutic surgery for resectable lesions.

Although fine-needle aspiration biopsy has been widely used in other countries, little enthusiasm existed in the United States for the procedure until fairly recently. Increased clinical acceptance of cytologic diagnosis has led to widespread use of the technique in this country, particularly in the past two decades. Extensive experience with needle aspiration has shown it to be relatively simple for the radiologist and well tolerated by the patient.

LESION LOCALIZATION

Localization is the most critical aspect of the procedure and it should be performed with great care. Plain radiography, fluoroscopy,[10, 11, 25] ultrasonography (US),[6, 16, 19, 21, 23] and computed tomography (CT)[4, 6, 14, 27] have all been used for localization of retroperitoneal masses. The choice of modality is much

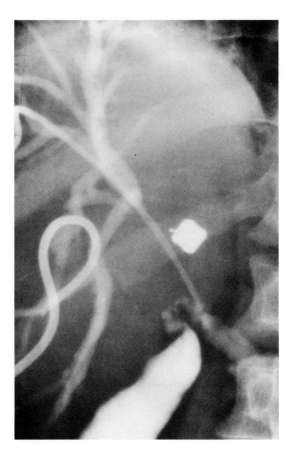

FIG 5–1.
Cholangiogram in a patient with a mass obstructing the common hepatic duct. A 22-gauge Chiba needle is placed in the mass under fluoroscopic guidance.

less important than that it be employed accurately, however. Fluoroscopic guidance is one of the most readily available and least expensive techniques. Biplane or angled, movable, C-arm fluoroscopic capabilities also enhance localization. If neither is available, a rotational cradle-top table may be of value. Small deep lesions can be more accurately localized and biopsied with CT than with fluoroscopy.

Localization may be facilitated by the administration of contrast material by any of a number of routes. Percutaneous cholangiography (Fig 5–1),[25] endoscopic retrograde cholangiopancreatography,[7, 18] angiography,[24, 29] lymph-angiography,[11, 12, 26] and excretory and antegrade pyelography[2] have all been used in conjunction with fine-needle aspiration biopsy.

BIOPSY TECHNIQUE

Only fine needles, 22- or 23-gauge, should be used with a transabdominal approach. Cytologic material can easily be obtained with any of the fine-needle types. Histologic material can also be obtained on occasion with a Chiba needle. However, the Greene,[20] Franseen,[1] Turner,[28] Sure-cut, and Rotex[22] needles are all commercially available in fine gauges and are designed to maximize the probability of obtaining a small tissue core. Use of larger gauge needles with the transabdominal approach is potentially associated with a greater chance of complications, including tumor seeding along the needle tract.[14, 15] If a posterior approach is used and the peritoneum is not traversed, a larger gauge needle can be used with greater confidence.

The procedure can be performed on an outpatient or inpatient basis. Patient preparation is minimal. A fast from midnight is often ordered if contrast material is to be administered. Premedication is not routinely administered, except for pediatric or apprehensive patients. Some patients may require administration of a relaxant or analgesic during the procedure.

Once the lesion is localized fluoroscopically, the intended needle path is determined. Major blood vessels, for example, the aorta and inferior vena cava,

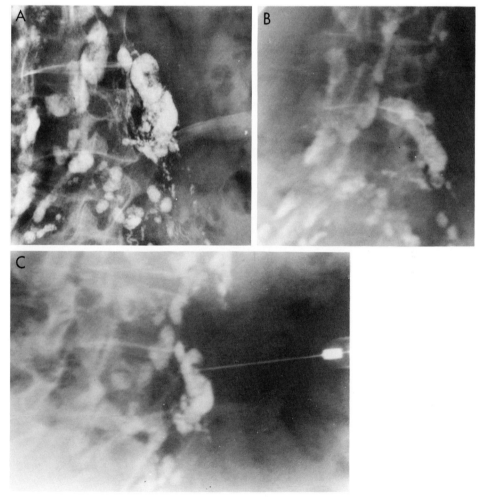

FIG 5–2.
Lymphangiogram. **A,** peripheral filling defect in a left common iliac lymph node in a patient with cervical carcinoma. **B,** tip of needle in the area of the filling defect. **C,** steep oblique film reveals needle tip across a suspicious area of the lymph node.

should be avoided if possible. If biplane or C-arm fluoroscopy is used, the lesion and its depth should also be identified in the lateral plane. The needle entrance site is chosen and marked. The skin is cleansed with antiseptic solution and draped. Local anesthesia is obtained in the dermis and subcutaneous tissue. A small dermatomy is made in the skin to facilitate needle placement. Needle placement should be performed along a vertical course with hub and the tip superimposed if possible (see Fig 5–1). Because of the flexibility of fine-needles, withdrawal and realignment may be necessary if the first placement is faulty, as the needle cannot be redirected by application of pressure on the hub. Patient respiration should be suspended during needle placement, which can be performed in small increments with frequent intermittent fluoroscopic checks.

Correct depth of the needle tip can be confirmed on the lateral view with biplane capacity (Fig 5–2). Several passes can be made in the lesion with a fine-needle, sampling from different regions by slight variations in needle angulation.

A tandem needle technique can also be used,[4] which potentially facilitates the ease and speed of the procedure. Initial placement is made with a Chiba needle, which remains in place as a guide for subsequent needle passes (see Fig 5–1). These can be made swiftly along the marker needle path, using a slightly different angulation if desired (Fig 5–3). The initial needle is then aspirated for an additional biopsy sample on withdrawal. This technique can also be used with US or CT localization. The coaxial[13] and modified coaxial[30] techniques can also be applied to retroperitoneal aspiration biopsy with fluoroscopic guidance.

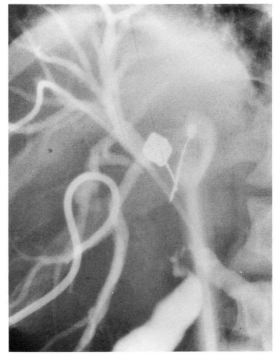

FIG 5–3.
A second biopsy needle (Rotex) is placed in a different site of the mass using a tandem technique.

The aspirated material is extruded onto slides that are promptly immersed and fixed for cytologic Papanicolaou examination. Any tissue core is placed in formalin for histologic evaluation. If abscess is a diagnostic consideration, cultures should also be obtained.

After the procedure, the patient's vital signs are monitored closely for three to four hours. Outpatients are asked to remain in the department for this period of time and then discharged in the company of a reliable person.

CONTRAINDICATIONS

As with fine-needle aspiration biopsy of the lung, most contraindications to aspiration biopsy of the abdomen are relative. Abnormal bleeding values should be corrected before the procedure, if possible. Aspiration can be performed on patients undergoing therapy with heparin, if the drug is discontinued four to six hours prior to the procedure. As controlled respiration is needed, uncooperative patients or those with uncontrollable coughs may not be candidates for fine-needle biopsy. Suitability must be determined on an individual basis.

Suspected vascular lesions can be biopsied with fine needles. Close monitoring of the patient's vital signs is important after the procedure. Suspected echinococcal cysts should not be aspirated because of the risk of an anaphylactic reaction and the potential of seeding the peritoneal cavity with daughter cysts.

SPECIAL CONSIDERATIONS

Pancreas

Pancreatic carcinoma is a relatively common malignancy and it is the fourth leading cause of death from cancer in men and the fifth most common in women.[17] Exploratory laparotomy is still frequently used for diagnostic purposes in conjunction with needle or wedge biopsy, despite suspected unresectability of the tumor. The benefit of percutaneous needle biopsy is obvious, if surgery can be avoided.

Fluoroscopic localization of a pancreatic mass can be assisted by opacification of the duodenal loop with barium or of the common bile duct by transhepatic[25] or endoscopic[7] cholangiography. Angiography can also be used as a guide.[24, 29]

The safety of percutaneous pancreatic biopsy is documented by Freeny and Lawson,[8] who described two minor complications in 219 cases. More serious complications have been reported, however. One case of tumor seeding occurred along the tract,[5] and one patient died from fulminant necrotizing pancreatitis[3] after fine-needle aspiration biopsy. The method of localization seems to be the most important factor in determining the rate of accuracy of percutaneous pancreatic aspiration biopsy. Endoscopic retrograde cholangiopancreatography and CT have the highest associated accuracy rates at 96%, followed by US and angiography both at 69%. Transhepatic cholangiography provides the lowest rate of accuracy, at 52%.[8]

Lymph Nodes

Percutaneous lymph node biopsy with fine needles can enhance the diagnostic accuracy of lymphangiography. The latter procedure is associated with a 5% to 10% occurrence of false-positive and 10% to 20% false-negative diagnoses.[31] Fine-needle aspiration biopsy is only helpful in reducing the rate of false-negative diagnoses.

After lymphangiographic opacification of the iliac and retroperitoneal nodes, transabdominal fine-needle aspiration can be performed under fluoroscopic guidance (see Fig 5–2). The preferred site of biopsy of a presumed metastatic defect due to carcinoma is just within the margin of the defect. The site of biopsy in presumed lymphomatous nodes is less critical due to the more diffuse nature of the disease.[32]

Adequate specimens from percutaneous fine-needle lymph node biopsy are obtained in approximately 80% of cases.[26] The yield of biopsy is greater in metastatic epithelial tumors than in lymphoma, with diagnosis established in 85% and 50% respectively.[31]

Urinary Tract

Fine-needle aspiration biopsy can be performed with a transabdominal approach on renal and ureteric lesions.[9] Opacification of the kidneys and collecting systems is accomplished with antegrade or retrograde pyelography or angiography.[25] A larger needle can be used with a posterior or posterolateral approach. In one small series, the correct diagnosis of malignancy was made in all nine patients who underwent biopsy by translumbar approach.[25]

CONCLUSION

Percutaneous aspiration biopsy of retroperitoneal masses can be safely performed with fluoroscopic guidance. A transabdominal approach should be used only with fine needles. A posterior approach that does not encroach on the peritoneal cavity can be used with fine or larger gauge needles. A variety of means of contrast administration are available and enhance the accuracy of the procedure.

REFERENCES

1. Ballard GL, Boyd WR: A specially designed cutting aspiration needle for lung biopsy. *AJR* 1978; 130:899–903.
2. Barbaric ZL, MacIntosh PK: Periureteral thin-needle aspiration biopsy. *Urol Radiol* 1981; 2:181–185.
3. Evans WK, et al: Fatal necrotizing pancreatitis following fine-needle aspiration biopsy of the pancreas. *Radiology* 1982; 141:61–62.
4. Ferrucci JT Jr, Wittenberg J: CT biopsy of abdominal tumors: Aids for lesion localization. *Radiology* 1978; 129:739–744.
5. Ferrucci JT Jr, et al: Malignant seeding of the tract after thin-needle aspiration biopsy. *Radiology* 1979; 130:345–346.

6. Ferrucci JT Jr, et al: Diagnosis of abdominal malignancy by radiologic fine-needle aspiration biopsy. *AJR* 1980; 134:323–330.
7. Freeny PC, Kidd R, Ball TJ: ERCP-guided percutaneous fine needle pancreatic biopsy. *West J Med* 1980; 132:283–287.
8. Freeny PC, Lawson TL: Adenocarcinoma of the pancreas, in Freeny PC, Lawson TL (eds): *Radiology of the Pancreas.* New York, Springer-Verlag, 1982, pp 397–496.
9. Freiman DB, et al: Thin-needle biopsy in the diagnosis of ureteral obstruction with malignancy. *Cancer* 1978; 42:714–716.
10. Goldstein H, Zornoza J, Wallace S: Percutaneous fine-needle aspiration biopsy of pancreatic and other abdominal masses. *Radiology* 1977; 123:319–322.
11. Gothlin JH: Post-lymphographic percutaneous fine-needle biopsy of lymph nodes guided by fluoroscopy. *Radiology* 1976; 120:205–207.
12. Gothlin JH, MacIntosh PK: Interventional radiology in the assessment of the retroperitoneal lymph nodes. *Radiol Clin North Am* 1979; 17:461–473.
13. Greene RF: Transthoracic needle aspiration, in Athanasoulis CA, et al (eds): *Interventional Radiology.* Philadelphia, WB Saunders Co, 1982, pp 587–634.
14. Haaga JR: New techniques for CT-guided biopsies. *AJR* 1979; 133:633–641.
15. Haaga RJ, Vanek J: Computed tomographic-guided liver biopsy using the Menghini needle. *Radiology* 1979; 133:405–408.
16. Hancke S, Holm HH, Koch F: Ultrasonically guided percutaneous fine-needle biopsy of the pancreas. *Surg Gynecol Obstet* 1975; 140:361–364.
17. Hermann RE, Cooperman AM: Current concepts in cancer: Cancer of the pancreas. *N Engl J Med* 1979; 301:482–485.
18. Ho CS, et al: Percutaneous fine-needle aspiration biopsy of the pancreas following endoscopic retrograde cholangiopancreatography. *Radiology* 1977; 125:351–352.
19. Holm HH, Als O, Gammelgaard J: Percutaneous aspiration and biopsy procedures under ultrasound visualization. *Clin Diag Ultrasound* 1979; 1:137.
20. Isler RJ, et al: Tissue core biopsy of abdominal tumors with a 22 gauge cutting needle. *AJR* 1981; 136:725–728.
21. Mets T, et al: Sonically guided renal biopsy. *J Clin Ultrasound* 1979; 7:190–191.
22. Nordenstrom B: New instruments for biopsy. *Radiology* 1975; 117:474–475.
23. Nosher JL, Plafker J: Fine-needle aspiration of the liver with ultrasound guidance. *Radiology* 1980; 136:177–180.
24. Oscarson J, Stormby N, Sundgren R: Selected angiography in fine-needle aspiration cytodiagnosis of gastric and pancreatic tumors. *Acta Radiol* 1972; 12:737–748.
25. Pereiras RM, et al: Fluoroscopically guided thin-needle aspiration biopsy of the abdomen and retroperitoneum. *AJR* 1978; 131:197–202.
26. Prando A, et al: Lymphangiography in staging of carcinoma of the prostate. The potential value of percutaneous lymph node biopsy. *Radiology* 1979; 131:641–645.
27. Stephenson TF, et al: Evaluation of contrast markers for CT aspiration biopsy. *AJR* 1979; 133:1097–1100.
28. Turner AF, Sargent EN: Percutaneous pulmonary needle biopsy. *AJR* 1968; 104:846–850.
29. Tylen V, et al: Percutaneous biopsy of carcinoma of the pancreas guided by angiography. *Surg Gynecol Obstet* 1976; 142:737–739.
30. vanSonnenberg E, et al: Percutaneous biopsy of difficult mediastinal, hilar and pulmonary lesions by computed tomographic guidance and a modified coaxial technique. *Radiology* 1983; 148:300–302.
31. Wallace S, Jing BS, Zornoza J: Lymphangiography in the determination of the extent of metastatic carcinoma: The potential value of percutaneous lymph node biopsy. *Cancer* 1977; 39(suppl):706–718.
32. Zornoza J: Abdomen, in Zornoza J (ed): *Percutaneous Needle Biopsy.* Baltimore, Williams & Wilkins Co, 1981, pp 102–140.

6

Pancreatic Biopsy and Drainage Guided by Ultrasound and Computed Tomography

Janis G. Letourneau, M.D.
Morteza K. Elyaderani, M.D.

Ultrasound (US) and computed tomography (CT) can provide target localization for lesions within the pancreas. Biopsy of solid or complex lesions within the pancreas can be accomplished with an anterior or more posterior approach. Drainage of pancreatic and peripancreatic guide collections requires precise localization that is often best provided with CT.

BIOPSY OF SOLID PANCREATIC MASSES

Surgical treatment of adenocarcinoma of the pancreas continues to be unrewarding. At the time of diagnosis, 90% of the tumors are unresectable, and the potential for cure is extremely low. The five-year survival rate is 1% to 2%.[25, 29] The mean survival was eight months in a series of patients treated for obstructive jaundice secondary to unresectable adenocarcinoma of the pancreas.[9] Postoperative mortality was 6% in the same series. Biopsy of a pancreatic mass with wedge resection or with a large-bore cutting needle, such as the Vim-Silverman needle, during laparotomy is inaccurate and is associated with a high morbidity and some mortality.[29] Serious postoperative complications related to the biopsy are hemorrhage, pancreatitis, fistula formation, and tumor-seeding.[23]

The majority of complications of intraoperative biopsy can be attributed to the large size of the needle used. Intraoperative biopsy using a fine needle, on the other hand, has demonstrated high accuracy and few or no complications. Accuracy with such methods has been reported to be 94.4%[6] and 96.5%.[15]

Percutaneous aspiration biopsy under the guidance of various imaging modalities, such as fluoroscopy in conjunction with arteriography or cholangiography, US, and CT, has been reported to allow accurate diagnosis in 75% to 85% of patients undergoing biopsy.[18, 26, 35] A combined approach with endoscopic retrograde cholangiopancreatography (ERCP) and pancreatic cytologic analysis plays an important role in diagnosis of pancreatic cancer.[29]

Method of Localization

Reliable diagnosis by percutaneous fine-needle aspiration depends on accurate localization. Fluoroscopy alone is not adequate for localization unless accompanied by another more invasive technique such as angiography, transhepatic cholangiography, or retrograde cholangiopancreatography (Fig 6–1).[36, 37]

Ultrasonography offers a rapid and simple method of localizing pancreatic masses (Fig 6–2). However, the pancreas may be obscured by overlying intestinal gas and the surrounding structures and viscera may not be seen as clearly as they are with CT. Generally, pancreatic tumors, primarily adenocarcinomas and islet cell neoplasms, are hypoechoic in nature; rarely they are hyperechoic in character. Because of technical limitations, such as overlying intestinal gas or patient obesity, the size of detectable lesions is variable. Lesions in the pancreas, particularly in the pancreatic head, are often associated with biliary and pancreatic ductal dilatation. In the setting of such ductal dilation careful search

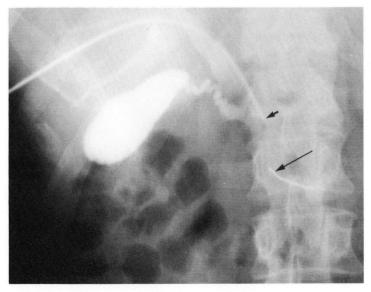

FIG 6–1.
Fine-needle aspiration of mass in the pancreatic head under fluoroscopic guidance. The fine needle *(long arrow)* is inserted along the common duct in the area of obstruction. Contrast material is injected to demonstrate the biliary system prior to aspiration. The tip of the guidewire is in the proximal common duct *(short arrow)*.

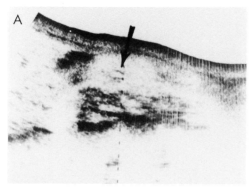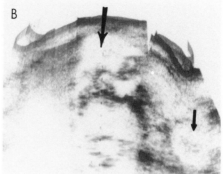

FIG 6–2.
A, longitudinal localization of a pancreatic mass by B-mode scanning *(arrow).* **B,** transverse localization of the same pancreatic mass *(large arrow).* The left kidney is also noted *(small arrow).*

for a focal mass should be made. Some pancreatic tumors will not be optimally
visualized by US preoperatively. Despite this situation, intraoperative sonography can be of value in localization of the focal abnormality and for planning
the therapeutic approach.[5, 27, 28]

Computed tomography is also a good method for localizing pancreatic neoplasms (Fig 6–3). It additionally provides considerable information regarding
nearby structures and the possibility of local and distant spread of malignancy.
It, unlike US, is not as adversely affected by adjacent bowel gas or patient
obesity. However, it does not allow for continuous monitoring of needle position during biopsy as is possible with fluoroscopy or US.

Both US and CT are sensitive in detecting pancreatic masses and can therefore be used with confidence for localization for fine-needle aspiration. Small
masses, measuring 1 to 2 cm in diameter, cannot be consistently detected with
either technique. A review of the recent literature reveals the overall accuracy
of US and CT to be 89% and 85%, respectively, for pancreatic mass detection,
with a true-positive rate of accuracy of 88% and 87%, respectively.[22]

Biopsy by Ultrasonographic or Computed Tomographic Guidance

The patient should fast for four to five hours before US-guided biopsy. The
patient is placed in a supine position, and the pancreatic mass is evaluated in

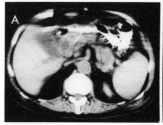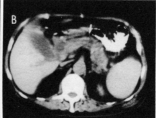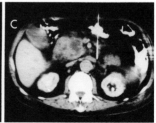

FIG 6–3.
Computed tomography shows a large mass in the pancreatic head. **A,** needle tip is in the mass in
the pancreatic head. **B,** needle tip near the body of the pancreas. **C,** needle tip is adjacent to the left
renal vein, improperly positioned.

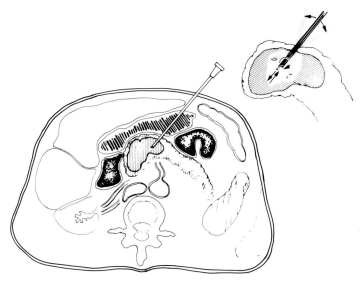

FIG 6–4.
Fine-needle aspiration of pancreatic mass avoiding puncture of the liver. It is not necessary to avoid the liver when biopsying the pancreas. Doing so usually increases the length of the needle tract.

two planes, transverse and longitudinal. The biopsy site is selected and the shortest possible route to the mass that avoids major blood vessels is chosen (Fig 6–4). Some organs, such as the stomach, bowel, and liver, may be traversed during biopsy with a fine caliber needle, but the spleen should not (Fig 6–5). The depth from the skin to the mass and the angle of approach are determined. Suspension of breathing in mid-inspiration minimizes dislodgement of the needle. Though static B-mode scanning with a biopsy transducer can be

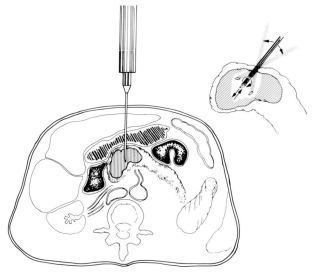

FIG 6–5.
Fine-needle aspiration of a pancreatic mass. Note that the needle passes through the liver and stomach.

used for percutanous biopsy of pancreatic masses, dynamic scanning with or without a biopsy transducer or adaptation is preferable. The latter equipment allows continuous visualization of the needle during placement and facilitates redirection of the needle if this is necessary (Fig 6–6).

Computed tomographic guidance for percutaneous aspiration biopsy of solid pancreatic masses is also valuable. Biopsy is usually performed from an anterior approach, but rarely may be performed from a posterior approach with the patient in a prone position. The biopsy site should be marked and the biopsy performed with the patient in suspended mid-inspiration. The patient should be allowed to breathe quietly while the needle tip position is checked by additional scans. Tandem or coaxial needle placement will maximize optimal needle localization.

Complications

Complications of pancreatic biopsy are directly related to the size of the needle and the number of biopsy attempts. With large needles the complication rate is reported to be between 2.7% and 20%, and the rate of associated mortality ranges from 1.5% to 3.8%.[8, 23, 32] Complications such as pancreatitis, hemorrhage, and fistula formation may occur after biopsy with large needles. Such complications are reduced significantly with use of a fine needle. A fine needle may pass through a variety of intraperitoneal and extraperitoneal viscera without complication during percutaneous aspiration, as its site of entry into the viscera appears to seal off immediately after its removal.

However, infection is possible even with fine-needle aspiration biopsy. Prophylactic antibiotics can be given to patients with a poor overall condition and

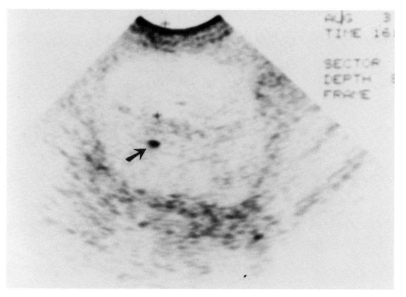

FIG 6–6.
Transverse sector scan of a large pancreatic mass shows the needle tip in the central portion of the mass *(arrow).*

to those with obstructive jaundice. They may be discontinued 24 hours after fine-needle aspiration if no further need is identified. The case of a patient in whom gram-negative sepsis developed following fine-needle aspiration biopsy has been reported.[14] It is assumed that intestine anterior to the pancreas was entered by the aspirating needle, resulting in bacteremia. If purulent material is aspirated from a pancreatic mass, appropriate antibiotic therapy should be given immediately, as peritonitis after fine-needle aspiration of an unsuspected abscess has been reported.[31] Surgical or percutaneous abscess drainage must then be considered.

A risk of percutaneous needle aspiration of malignant masses is dissemination of tumor cells along the needle tract or through lymph or blood. Experimental investigation has shown tumor cells along the needle tract, but not within the blood vessels or efferent lymph.[11] Malignant seeding of the tract after aspiration biopsy with a 22-gauge needle has been reported,[13] and cutaneous seeding has been described following fine-needle aspiration of a pancreatic cancer.[35]

ASPIRATION AND DRAINAGE OF PANCREATIC FLUID COLLECTIONS

Diagnostic aspiration biopsy can be performed under US or CT guidance for any apparently fluid-filled pancreatic mass. Precise localization is the key to a successful procedure. The procedure is performed similarly to that of percutaneous biopsy of solid pancreatic masses. If the fluid collection proves to be purulent, drainage can be immediately initiated (Fig 6–7).

Fluid-filled pancreatic masses are readily detected by US and CT. They include more common entities, abscess and pseudocyst, and also less common

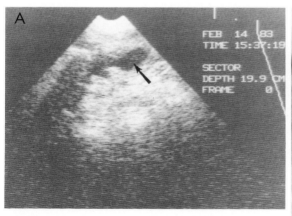
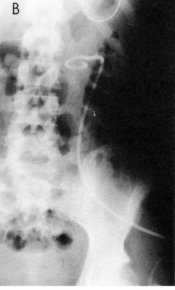

FIG 6–7.
A, transverse sonogram shows a cystic mass with internal echoes *(arrow)* in the region of the pancreas. **B,** after pus was obtained by fine-needle aspiration, a pigtail catheter was inserted and the mass was drained.

entities, cystadenoma, cystadenocarcinoma, and hematoma. Percutaneous fine-needle aspiration may be useful in the diagnosis of all these processes[20]; percutaneous drainage may be therapeutic for abscess and pseudocyst. Sonographically, these fluid-filled pancreatic masses may not be distinguishable (Fig 6–8). Gas in a pancreatic abscess may be highly reflective; but in the absence of gas, abscess, pseudocyst, cystadenoma, cystadenocarcinoma, and hematoma may appear similarly, as primarily sonolucent structures with a variable amount of internal structure and echogenicity. On CT, differentiation of these masses may also be difficult. Although the presence of gas in an apparently fluid-filled pancreatic mass is essentially pathognomonic of an abscess,[10] its presence may reflect previous surgery or other intervention, as well as communication with bowel. An abscess without gas and an attenuation value more like soft tissue may alternately simulate a neoplasm.

Pancreatic Abscess

Pancreatic abscesses are collections of infected necrotic material lying within the pancreas or extending from the pancreas into the remainder of the retroperitoneum, lesser sac, and mesentery. It is the most serious complication of acute pancreatitis and is associated with a high mortality. It has been estimated that abscesses develop in 4% of all patients with pancreatitis and in approximately 40% of patients with hemorrhagic or necrotizing pancreatitis.[12] Survival from pancreatic abscess without drainage is uncommon and with external drainage is about 66%.[12] Early drainage is desirable.

Fluid collection within the pancreas is suggestive, but not diagnostic, of pancreatic abscess. If the fluid collection has gas within it, the diagnosis is more

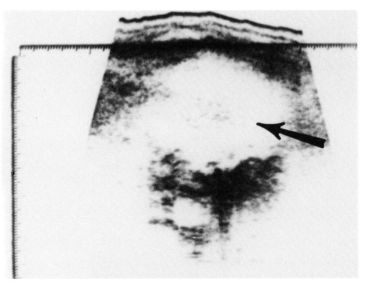

FIG 6–8.
A large cystic mass with internal echoes *(arrow)* is seen in the body of the pancreas. The mass was an infected pseudocyst.

likely. However, gas was detected in only 29% of pancreatic abscesses in one series.[12] In approximately one third of the patients, the abscesses are multiple or multiloculated. Ultrasonography and CT seem to be the primary imaging modalities for diagnosis of pancreatic abscess.

Because ileus often occurs in these patients, US may fail to adequately visualize the pancreas. However, it can be a valuable diagnostic tool, especially when used portably for patients in poor general condition. A fluid collection with internal echoes and poorly defined margins or irregular wall suggests the diagnosis. These sonographic criteria also may, however, be seen in the early stages of pseudocyst formation or with an infected pseudocyst. Computed tomography defines the features of pancreatic abscess as well, demonstrating a fluid collection of variable attenuation sometimes surrounded by an ill-defined or irregular wall. Gas bubbles may be readily appreciated if present. The preferred examination is CT, as it best defines the number and extension of abscesses into the surrounding regions.

Pancreatic Pseudocyst

The development of a pseudocyst is preceded by pancreatic inflammation, as seen in approximately 90% of the cases, or by trauma.[30] The cystic fluid contains pancreatic enzymes in high concentrations; the amylase level within the pseudocyst may range from 3 to 50 times the normal serum value. The fluid in the cyst originates from the acinar cells or directly from the pancreatic ducts.[10] This communication can be demonstrated by direct injection of contrast material into the cyst or by endoscopic retrograde pancreatography.[1] After a few weeks, the fluid within the pseudocyst and its associated inflammatory reaction induce the formation of a surrounding fibrous capsule.

Data from Bradley et al.[4] support a program of serial observations of early, uncomplicated pseudocysts in the hope of spontaneous resolution (Fig 6–9). A wide spectrum of complications has been reported in patients with untreated pseudocysts, including infection, rupture, and hemorrhage. If there is evidence of secondary infection or pseudocyst enlargement or if spontaneous resolution

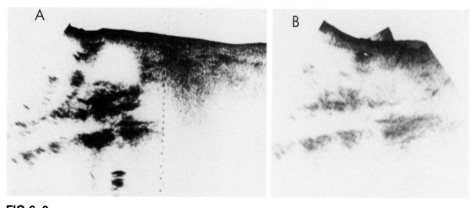

FIG 6–9.
A, longitudinal sonogram of a pancreatic pseudocyst after traumatic pancreatitis. **B,** longitudinal sonogram of the same patient shows resolution of the pseudocyst in three weeks.

has not occurred within four to seven weeks, the issue is complicated, however. Spontaneous regression of pseudocysts is reported to be as common as 25%.[3, 4, 7, 34] On the other hand, complications occurred twice as frequently as spontaneous resolution in an observation period of three to four weeks.[4]

Diagnostic Aspiration of Pancreatic Abscesses or Pseudocysts

Diagnostic percutaneous aspiration biopsy of pancreatic abscesses or pseudocysts can be performed with US or CT guidance. A fine needle should be used for the aspiration, as bowel may be intervening along the needle tract to the pancreas. Ultrasonographic guidance allows adequate localization for many pancreatic fluid collections and can be provided portably if needed. It may not provide as much information as CT, however, especially in the setting of potential percutaneous or surgical drainage.[20]

Ultrasonographic guidance for aspiration requires precise localization of the fluid collection in both longitudinal and transverse planes. Aspiration can be accomplished without or with the aid of a biopsy transducer. Guidance by CT can be used as the primary means of localization if percutaneous drainage is planned, as it provides more precise information regarding adjacent viscera. Whereas it is acceptable to traverse bowel for a diagnostic aspiration, it is not desirable to do so in the setting of percutaneous catheter drainage. Respiration

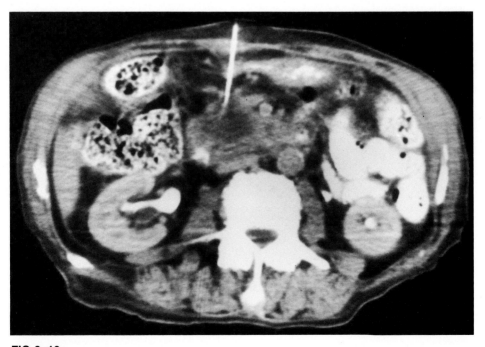

FIG 6–10.
Computed tomography during biopsy of a pancreatic carcinoma located in the head and proximal body of the pancreas. Biopsy was accomplished with a 22-gauge fine-needle using a tandem technique following fine-needle localization. Note the needle tract passes through the gastric antrum.

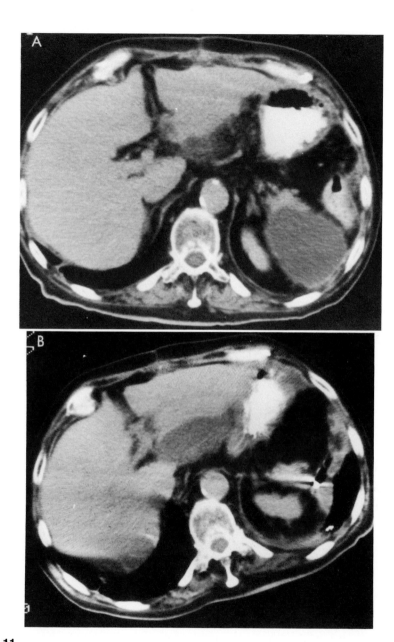

FIG 6–11.
A, a large pancreatic pseudocyst is seen on computed tomography adjacent to the upper pole of the left kidney. The patient has undergone a splenectomy. **B,** Computed tomographic scan at the same level as **A** following percutaneous catheter drainage of the pancreatic pseudocyst. Complete evacuation of that fluid collection is seen. An additional fluid collection is seen adjacent to the left lobe of the liver.

should be suspended in mid-inspiration for the needle placement and the aspiration, but can be resumed for confirmation of the needle position by US or CT.

Percutaneous Drainage of Pancreatic Abscesses and Pseudocysts

Needle or catheter drainage can be performed by a percutaneous route as either a temporizing or a potentially therapeutic maneuver. Catheter drainage rather than needle aspiration is preferred for abscesses in particular and must be done in conjunction with systemic antibiotic treatment. Guidance by CT is the ideal imaging modality for determining the catheter course, as it best defines the surrounding viscera and blood vessels, unless the location of the mass has already been defined and surrounding loops of bowel are known to be displaced away from the mass.

The intended path of the catheter must be planned with care. Computed tomography provides critical information regarding the location of nearby loops of bowel, the stomach, the liver, the spleen, the kidneys, and the inferior vena cava and aorta. A posterolateral approach will generally be the safest, as bowel loops tend to lie anteriorly (Fig 6–10). However, a mass may lie so close to the anterior abdominal wall that no bowel loops intervene. Under such circumstances an anterior approach can be used safely.

Following careful localization of an abscess or pseudocyst, catheter drainage can be accomplished by a variety of methods (Fig 6–11). A single-stick technique with a fine needle and 0.018-in. guidewire can be used. Alternatively, following fine-needle localization, a tandem approach using a larger needle and the Seldinger technique can be used. If the mass is relatively large and the intended tract direct, the Seldinger technique can be used at the onset without initial fine-needle localization.

Large series of this type of treatment have not been reported.[1, 2, 16, 17, 19, 21, 24, 33] Some fluid collections appear to completely resolve; others still require surgical drainage. However, needle or catheter drainge may provide adequate therapy or time to prepare and plan necessary surgery when this is not immediately desired or indicated.

CONCLUSION

Percutaneous aspiration biopsy of pancreatic masses can be performed with relative safety and ease with US and CT guidance. Therapeutic drainage of pancreatic fluid collections can be performed by needle aspiration or catheter placement. If a catheter is placed, CT usually provides the most accurate guidance for such drainage.

REFERENCES

1. Andersen BN, et al: The diagnosis of pancreatic cyst by endoscopic retrograde pancreatography and ultrasonic scanning. *Ann Surg* 1977; 183:286–289.

2. Barkin JS, et al: Therapeutic percutaneous aspiration of pancreatic pseudocysts. *Dig Dis Sci* 1981; 26:585–586.

3. Bradley EL, Clements JL: Spontaneous resolution of pancreatic pseudocysts. *Am J Surg* 1975; 129:23–28.

4. Bradley EL, Clements JL, Gonzalez AC: The natural history of pancreatic pseudocysts: A unified concept of management. *Am J Surg* 1979; 137:135–141.

5. Charboneau JW, et al: Intraoperative real time ultrasonographic localization of pancreatic insulinoma: Initial experience. *J Ultrasound Med* 1983; 2:251–254.

6. Christofferson P, Poll P: Preoperative pancreas aspiration biopsies. *Acta Pathol Microbiol Scand (suppl)* 1970; 212:28–29.

7. Czaja AJ, Fisher M, Martin GA: Spontaneous resolution of pancreatic masses (pseudocysts?): Development and disappearance after acute alcoholic pancreatitis. *Arch Intern Med* 1975; 135:558–562.

8. Dekker A, Lloyd JC: Fine-needle aspiration biopsy in ampullary and pancreatic carcinoma. *Arch Surg* 1979; 114:592–596.

9. Dozois RR: Operative and nonoperative therapy for cancer of the pancreas. Presented at the 68th Annual Clinical Congress of the American College of Surgeons, Postgraduate Course 3, Diseases of the liver, biliary tract, and pancreas, Chicago, Oct 24–29, 1982.

10. Elliot DW: Pancreatic pseudocysts. *Surg Clin North Am* 1975; 55:339–362.

11. Engzell U, et al: Investigation of tumour spread in connection with aspiration biopsy. *Acta Radiol (Diagn) (Stockh)* 1971; 10:385–389.

12. Federle MP, et al: Computed tomography of pancreatic abscesses. *AJR* 1981; 136:879–882.

13. Ferrucci JT Jr, et al: Malignant seeding of the tract after thin-needle biopsy. *Radiology* 1979; 130:345–346.

14. Ferrucci JT Jr, et al: Diagnosis of abdominal malignancy by radiologic fine-needle aspiration biopsy. *AJR* 1980; 134:323–330.

15. Forsgren L, Oreil S: Aspiration cytology in carcinoma of the pancreas. *Surgery* 1973; 73:38–42.

16. Gerzof SB, et al: Percutaneous catheter drainage of abdominal abscesses guided by ultrasound and computed tomography. *AJR* 1979; 133:1–8.

17. Haaga JR, et al: Percutaneous CT-guided pancreatography and pseudocystography. *AJR* 1979; 132:829–830.

18. Hancke S, Holm HH, Koch F: Ultrasonically guided percutaneous fine-needle biopsy of the pancreas. *Surg Gynecol Obstet* 1975; 140:361.

19. Hancke S, Pedersen JF: Percutaneous puncture of pancreatic cysts guided by ultrasound. *Surg Gynecol Obstet* 1976; 142:551–552.

20. Hill MC, et al: The role of percutaneous aspiration in the diagnosis of pancreatic abscess. *AJR* 1983; 141:1035–1038.

21. Karlson KB, et al: Percutaneous drainage of pancreatic pseudocysts and abscesses. *Radiology* 1982; 142:619–624.

22. Kurtz AB, Goldberg BB: in Goldberg BB (ed): *Abdominal Ultrasonography,* ed 2. New York, John Wiley and Sons, 1984, pp 163–206.

23. Lightwood R, Reber HA, Way LW: The risk and accuracy of pancreatic biopsy. *Am J Surg* 1976; 132:189–194.

24. MacErlean DP, Bryan PJ, Murphy JJ: Pancreatic pseudocyst: Management by ultrasonically guided aspiration. *Gastrointest Radiol* 1980; 5:255–257.

25. McCormack LR, Seat SG, Strum WB: Pancreatic carcinoma: Survival following detection by ultrasonic scanning. *JAMA* 1977; 238:240.

26. Oscarson J, Stormby N, Sundgren R: Selective angiography in fine-needle aspiration cyto-diagnosis of gastric and pancreatic tumors. *Acta Radiol (Diagn) (Stockh)* 1972; 12:737.

27. Plainfosse MC, Merran S: Work in progress: Intraoperative ultrasound. *Radiology* 1983; 147:829–832.
28. Rifkin MD, Weiss SM: Intraoperative sonography: Identification of nonpalpable pancreatic masses. *J Ultrasound Med* 1984; 3:409–411.
29. Sahel J: Pancreatic cancer: ERCP, in *Early Diagnosis of Pancreatic Cancer.* New York, Igaku-Shoin, 1980, pp 118–139.
30. Sankaran S, Walt AJ: The natural and unnatural history of pancreatic pseudo-cysts. *Br J Surg* 1975; 62:37–44.
31. Schnyder PA, Candardjis G, Anderegg A: Peritonitis after thin-needle aspiration biopsy of an abscess. *AJR* 1981; 137:1271–1272.
32. Schultz NJ, Sanders RJ: Evaluation of pancreatic biopsy. *Ann Surg* 1954; 139:403–408.
33. Schwerk WB: Ultrasonically guided percutaneous puncture and analysis of aspirated material of cystic pancreatic lesions. *Digestion* 1981; 21:184–192.
34. Slovis TL, VonBerg VJ, Mikelic V: Sonography in the diagnosis and management of pancreatic pseudocysts and effusions in childhood. *Radiology* 1980; 135:153–155.
35. Smith FP, et al: Cutaneous seeding of pancreatic cancer by skinny-needle aspiration biopsy. *Arch Intern Med* 1980; 140:55.
36. Tao LC, et al: Percutaneous fine-needle biopsy of the pancreas: Cytodiagnosis of pancreatic carcinoma. *Acta Cytol* 1978; 22:215–220.
37. Tylen U, et al: Percutaneous biopsy of carcinoma of the pancreas guided by an-giography. *Surg Gynecol Obstet* 1976; 142:737–739.

Percutaneous Biopsy of Kidneys and Adrenals and Drainage of Nephric and Perinephric Fluid Collections

Janis G. Letourneau, M.D.
Morteza K. Elyaderani, M.D.

Percutaneous biopsy and drainage techniques are valuable in the diagnosis and treatment of renal masses and perinephric fluid collections. Guidance for these procedures can be provided by fluoroscopy, ultrasound (US), or computed tomography (CT), with these imaging modalities often being complementary to one another.

DIAGNOSTIC APPROACH TO CYSTIC RENAL MASSES

Cystic renal masses are common, with benign simple renal cysts seen in approximately 50% of all patients over the age of 55 years. These must be differentiated from neoplastic and inflammatory processes. Therefore, when a renal mass is detected radiographically, it is first necessary to establish whether it is cystic or solid in nature. If the mass is discovered by intravenous (IV) urography and nephrotomography, it can be further evaluated by US to better determine its character. If sonographic criteria for simple cysts are fulfilled, no further diagnostic evaluation is warranted.[55] If the criteria are not met, cyst aspiration with laboratory evaluation usually provides a definitive diagnosis, and invasive procedures such as angiography may be obviated. Nonsurgical treatment of renal cysts can also be undertaken if desired. When the mass is solid, further diagnostic studies, such as radionuclide scanning, CT, or angiography, should be performed.

Ultrasonography

The classic diagnostic sonographic criteria for simple renal cysts are (1) absence of internal echogenicity, (2) smooth, sharply defined walls, and (3) acoustic enhancement beyond the posterior wall[55] (Fig 7–1). Sonography is usually the diagnostic modality of choice for evaluation of a patient with a known renal mass or one in whom a renal mass has been detected incidentally during IV urography or abdominal CT. Computed tomography may be used rather than US, if other indications for the examination exist. Sometimes US or CT criteria for simple renal cysts are not met; in these cases angiography or cyst puncture with cystogram should be performed to document the benign character of the mass.

At first glance these diagnostic criteria may seem simple, but when they are applied in practice, numerous pitfalls are encountered. Simple cysts, especially when small, may lack a sharp, smooth posterior wall and often contain internal artifactual echoes. The presence of artifactual echoes is affected to a significant degree by the beam width of the transducer. Thus if the beam width is greater than the diameter of the cyst, echoes from adjacent structures may appear to be within the cyst.[10] In general, the highest frequency focused transducer that

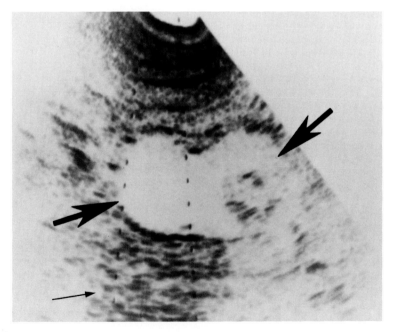

FIG 7–1.
Transverse sonogram of a simple cyst with well-demarcated posterior wall and acoustic enhancement. Cyst *(left large arrow)*, kidney *(right large arrow)*, and acoustic enhancement *(small arrow)*.

will penetrate the patient should be used. Attention to technical details is also important with respect to the second criterion, sharply defined walls. Frequently, because of reverberation, the near wall will lack a smooth contour. This artifactual error can be eliminated by changing the gain or the direction from which the cyst is examined. Posterior acoustic enhancement should always be present, even with a small cyst. A firm and accurate diagnosis of simple renal cyst can be made with a reliability of 95% if all the ultrasonic criteria are fulfilled.[44]

Computed Tomography

Computed tomography has proven to be a reasonably accurate means of differentiating benign renal cysts from neoplasms. Sagel and associates[60] reported a diagnostic accuracy approaching 100%. Cyst walls are usually not detectable on CT images as structures distinct from the interiors. The interiors of benign cysts generally have a uniform attenuation value near that of water and do not change in appearance on contrast-enhanced scans. Attenuation values of small cysts are less reliable because volume averaging with normal renal tissue can raise them substantially (Fig 7–2). Thin-section CT is a potential solution to the problem of partial volume averaging. Attenuation densities slightly greater than those of normal renal parenchyma prior to contrast enhancement can be caused by blood within simple cysts or by necrotic neoplasms.

Angiography

Angiography may be needed to evaluate a cystic renal lesion if other procedures, such as US or cyst puncture, are not diagnostic. The angiographic characteristics of a benign renal cyst are as follows (Fig 7–3).
1. Spheric and crescentic displacement of interlobular and arcuate vessels around an avascular nonstaining mass.
2. Sharp demarcation between cyst and adjacent normally staining parenchyma in the capillary-nephrographic phase.

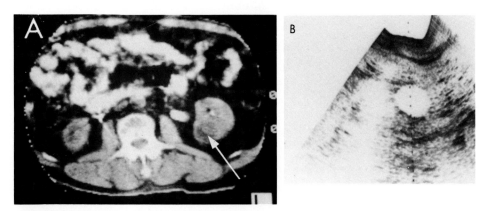

FIG 7–2.
A, computed tomographic scan of a renal cyst with a nonspecific appearance because of partial-volume averaging *(arrow)*. **B,** sonogram of the same patient shows features of a simple renal cyst.

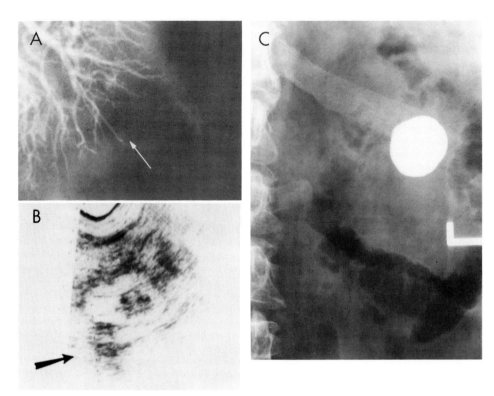

FIG 7–3.
A, selective renal arteriography shows an avascular mass *(arrow).* **B,** prone transverse sonogram shows cystic mass with acoustic through transmission *(arrow).* The wall of the cyst is not well seen. **C,** cystogram of the same patient following aspiration of cystic contents.

RENAL CYST ASPIRATION

A cystic renal mass may demonstrate thick, irregular, or calcified walls, septations, or internal echoes with sonographic examination. Such a cystic mass should undergo further diagnostic evaluation (Figs 7–4, 7–5, and 7–6), as should cysts with benign characteristics in the clinical setting of pain or microscopic hematuria (Fig 7–7). Additionally, any cystic mass that cannot be definitively evaluated by US because of technical considerations, including patient obesity, also warrants further evaluation. If on CT examination a cystic mass has an irregular shape, thick wall, or high or nonuniform attenuation value, US and cyst aspiration can be performed.[4, 12] Some authors think that certain CT qualities, such as a smooth wall, a relatively high precontrast density, and a homogenous postcontrast density, are characteristic of a benign cyst, despite hyperdensity.[73]

Fluoroscopic Guidance

With the patient in a prone position, a drip-infusion pyelogram is started to visualize the kidneys. The depth of the lesion must be determined by multidi-

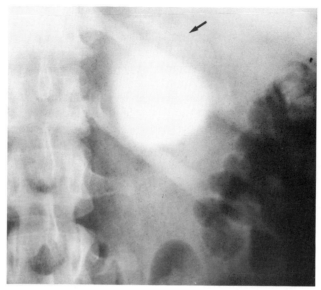

FIG 7–4.
Cystogram of a simple cyst with calcified wall *(arrow).*

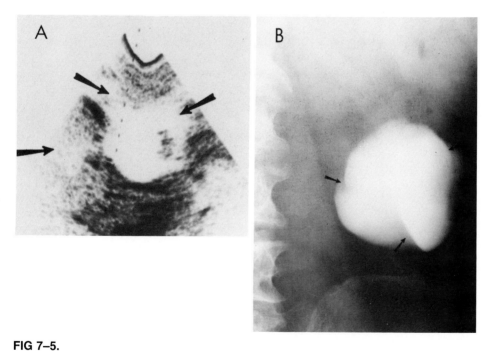

FIG 7–5.
A, transverse sonogram of a renal cyst shows irregularity of the wall *(arrow).* **B,** cystogram of the same patient shows septations of the cyst *(arrows).*

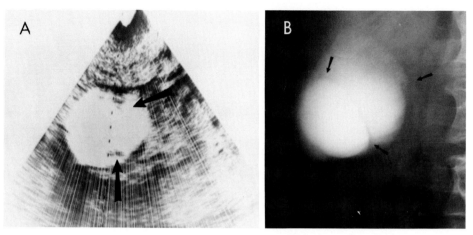

FIG 7–6.
A, transverse sonogram of renal cyst with internal septations *(arrows).* **B,** cystogram of the same patient shows multiple septations *(arrows).*

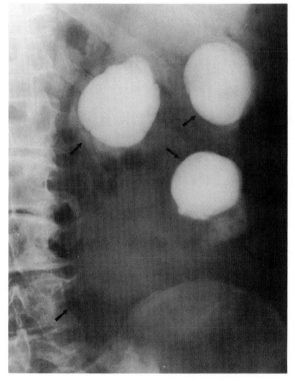

FIG 7–7.
Cystograms of five simple renal cysts *(arrows)* obtained after aspiration in a patient with hematuria.

rectional or biplane fluoroscopy or from the previously obtained nephrotomographic images.

Disadvantages of fluoroscopy-guided cyst aspiration are as follows.

1. Exposure of patient and operator to radiation.
2. Difficulty determining the depth and angle of approach if multidirectional or biplane fluoroscopy is not available.
3. Poor visualization of the cyst if it is small or if the patient is obese.

This means of localization was more popular in the past, but with the availability of newer imaging techniques, it is used less frequently.[42, 63] Sonographic localization is often preferred, especially in patients with renal insufficiency or contrast sensitivity.

Ultrasonography Guidance

With the patient in the prone position, longitudinal and transverse scans are performed through the kidney. Many different modes of US localization are available, but real-time sector or linear-array methods are currently the most popular. Aspiration can be performed without or with a transducer modified or specially designed for biopsy. If a real-time transducer is used, the entire shaft of the aspirating needle should be visualized during placement if possible. This requires that the needle path remains within the plane of the transducer sector. This task is facilitated, but not guaranteed, by a side arm attachment on the transducer for the needle or by a specialized biopsy transducer.

Computed Tomography Guidance

After the cyst has been localized on diagnostic scans, the entry site is selected and a metal marker is taped on the skin at that level. A repeat scan is then performed to verify the puncture site and allow for any necessary readjustments. The depth and angle of the puncture can be determined before the needle is inserted. Although CT is quite an accurate means of localization, it does not allow the continuous monitoring of needle position during placement that is possible with fluoroscopic and sonographic guidance.

Technique of Cyst Aspiration and Cystogram

After localization, the puncture is usually performed with a 22-gauge thin-walled needle coupled to polyethylene connecting tubing, a flexible system that permits movement of the needle during respiratory excursions. This flexibility is sacrificed when the various US biopsy transducers are employed. A portion of the calculated cyst volume is aspirated and the same volume of contrast (Renografin 60) is injected. Radiographs with the patient in the prone (Fig 7–8,A), supine (Fig 7–8,B), upright (Fig 7–8,C), decubitus (Fig 7–8,D), and occasionally Trendelenburg positions are then obtained. The resulting cystogram not only confirms that the cyst was entered and aspirated, but provides useful information about the cyst itself, such as its inner structure and walls. If there is question of extravasation of contrast material (Fig 7–9), a radiograph taken three to four hours after instillation of contrast into the cyst can be useful.

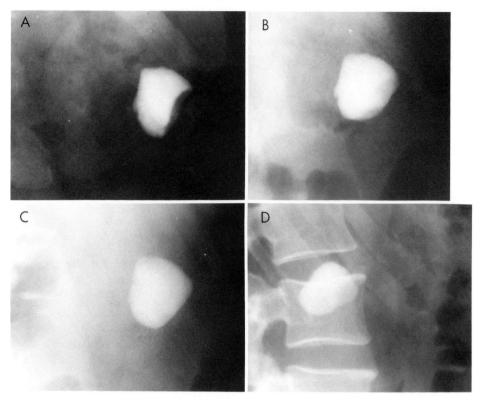

FIG 7–8.
Single-contrast cystogram obtained after cyst aspiration. Patient in prone **(A)**, supine **(B)**, upright **(C)**, and decubitus **(D)** positions.

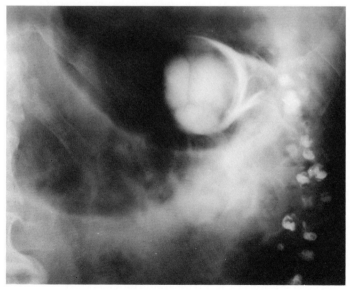

FIG 7–9.
Extravasation of contrast material after cystogram.

A double-contrast study can be performed if one desires better definition of the inner cyst wall (Fig 7–10). Approximately 25% of the estimated cyst volume is withdrawn and is replaced by equal amounts of air and contrast. Roentgenograms are obtained with the patient in the prone, supine, upright, decubitus, and Trendelenburg positions for further delineation of the inner wall.

Analysis of Aspirate

The characteristic features of an aspirate from a benign renal cyst are straw-colored fluid with low fat and protein content and negative cytologic findings. Clear fluid is not necessarily indicative of a benign process. If the aspirate is turbid or bloody, further evaluation must include culture and cytologic examination.

Complications of Cyst Puncture and Aspiration

Complications of renal cyst aspiration were studied in a survey of 5,674 cases reported by 84 institutions.[43] The overall incidence of significant complications was 1.4%, but was only 0.75% in institutions with extensive experience in the technique. The major complications of renal cyst puncture in order of frequency are perirenal hemorrhage, pneumothorax, infection, arteriovenous fistula, urinoma, and severe and prolonged hematuria. Rupture of the kidney, colon, and duodenum and development of bile peritonitis are uncommon complications. Minor complications such as transient gross hematuria, microhematuria, extravasation of contrast medium, pain, and fever occurred in approximately 10% of all patients, but were reported only at institutions undertaking routine follow-up. Flexible aspirating systems lessened the risk of major complications. An oblique approach to lesions in the upper poles of the kidneys using fluoroscopic or US guidance decreased the risk of pneumothorax compared with introduction of the needle through an US biopsy transducer. In

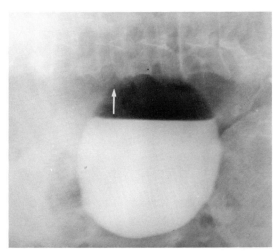

FIG 7–10.
Lateral decubitus view of a double-contrast study of simple cyst. Note smooth inner wall *(arrow).*

this series, the frequency of complications did not correlate with the number of puncture attempts, the gauge of puncture needle, or the completeness of evacuation.

ASPIRATION AND SCLEROSIS OF BENIGN RENAL CYSTS

Most simple benign cysts produce no symptoms and treatment is probably unnecessary. Occasionally, they cause pain, hydronephrosis,[29, 51] hypertension,[3] and polycythemia.[38] Treatment by simple aspiration is often temporary because of reaccumulation of fluid in 30% to 78%.[58, 62] Simple aspiration may, however, be used as a clinical trial to alleviate symptoms. If they are reduced, permanent treatment can be attempted by sclerosis of the cyst.

This issue is a controversial one, however. Dean[15] reported long-term cyst decompression after simple aspiration in 15 patients. Although his results have not been consistently duplicated, decrease in cyst size after simple aspiration has been reported occasionally by others.[20, 47, 54] Wahlquist and Grumstedt[69] described cyst decompression after aspiration alone in 24 of 52 lesions, including complete disappearance in 13 patients, with a mean follow-up time of 2.8 years.

Sclerosis of benign renal cysts can be traced to Fish,[20] who used a 50% dextrose solution as the sclerosing agent. Quinine-urea, cholohydrolactate,[45] 50% glucose,[27] and phenol[32] were also used as sclerosing agents. Vestby[65] subsequently reported success in diminishing renal cyst size in 18 patients following local instillation of iophendylate (Pantopaque). A controlled study later demonstrated a lower recurrence rate following sclerosis of simple cysts with iophendylate (56 cases) than that following simple aspiration (15 cases).[57]

Sclerosis of Renal Cysts with Iophendylate

After localization of the cyst by fluoroscopy, US, or CT, approximately 25% of the estimated volume is aspirated.[48] Approximately 80% of the aspirated fluid is replaced by Renografin 60. A film is obtained to confirm that the fluid is in the cyst and not in the renal collecting system. If vascular structures are visualized during the injection of Renografin 60, iophendylate should not be injected so as to avoid the risk of pulmonary embolism. Iophendylate is then injected according to cyst volume. Typically, about 3 ml of iophendylate is required for cysts less than 100 ml in volume, with approximately 6 ml required for those greater than 300 ml in volume. The total volume instilled into the cyst should be slightly less than the amount initially aspirated to minimize the risk of extravasation.

Iophendylate is thought to cause a local proliferative inflammatory reaction due to its free fatty acid component.[64] It has been noted to cause some fever and local pain following sclerosis of a renal cyst.[66] While the long-term effect of locally injected iophendylate may be speculative, it has been associated with adjacent marked chronic inflammatory change.[65] Clear demonstration of long-term safety for renal or perirenal tissues that might be so injected is unavailable from animal studies or clinical experience. The absorption of iophendylate from tissues is as slow as 1 ml per year; consequently toxicity to other organ systems, particularly the central nervous system (CNS) should be low.[53] Although Vestby[65] was the first to report on this technique, Raskin et al.[58] reported 68% of all renal cysts treated with intracystic iophendylate showed a significant decrease in size (50%), whereas only 13% managed without iophendylate showed a similar change. Ross et al.[59] also reported cyst regression in nine of 13 patients treated with local instillation of iophendylate. It can be concluded from these reports that intracystic iophendylate can produce a more significant decrease in cyst volume than can be explained by puncture alone.

Sclerosis of Renal Cysts With Alcohol

Alcohol can also be used as a sclerosing agent for simple renal cysts. A technique for this treatment was described by Bean and was used to treat 34 cysts in 29 patients.[6] Under US guidance with a standard diagnostic transducer, the renal masses were punctured with an 18-gauge, thin-walled arteriographic needle. Using the Seldinger method, a 4.6 French (F) 30-cm pigtail polyethylene catheter was advanced into the cystic mass. The fluid was aspirated and a double-contrast cystogram was performed. The contrast medium and air were then removed through the indwelling catheter. Masses that met the criteria of a benign cyst, clear fluid on aspiration, and smooth internal wall on cystogram were injected with 95% ethanol.

Instillation of 12% or more of the estimated cyst volume with 95% ethanol was adequate to prevent re-formation of the cyst. A smaller replacement (3.7%) was thought to be the cause of the one failure in the series. Volume replacement of 25% is probably ideal, since it will maximize contact of the sclerosing agent with cells in the cyst lining, but not create enough pressure to cause extravasation. The 95% ethanol is allowed to remain in place for ten to 20 minutes and then is removed through the pigtail catheter. Free flow of fluid in and out of the indwelling pigtail catheter was documented before alcohol is injected. If not present, no therapy was attempted.

Complications encountered in this series were no greater than in cyst aspiration alone. The patients were followed up by US from three to 30 months. There was one recurrence at three months.[6]

RENAL ABSCESSES

Renal abscesses occur in patients of all ages but are most common in young adults and are more frequent in males than females. Hematogenous spread from an extraurinary site or retrograde ascent from the lower urinary tract is the usual mode of development of a renal carbuncle. Predisposing conditions include the presence of skin furuncles, diabetes, pregnancy, prostatism, and neurogenic bladder.[37] Staphylococci have been the most common causative organisms in the past; however, recent reports indicate that gram-negative organisms now predominate.[19, 36]

The patient often has pain and tenderness localized to the flank, but the clinical signs may be vague. In patients with a subacute or chronic course, the diagnosis becomes much more difficult.

The radiographic evaluation of a suspected renal abscess begins with IV pyelography and nephrotomography. Since the radiographic findings are non-specific, however, additional diagnostic tests are often necessary. Ultrasonography is useful in revealing the size, number, and location of renal abscesses, as well as possible extension of renal abscess into the perinephric space.[50] It also may suggest the diagnosis.[22, 25] Typically, renal abscesses are echo-free masses with irregular thick walls. Internal echoes are sometimes present. An infected cyst, tumor with central necrosis, or hematoma may demonstrate similar findings.

If US is not diagnostic for technical reasons, such as the size of the patient or the presence of overlying bony structures, a CT scan should be done.[46] The CT can characterize an intrarenal fluid collection and also demonstrate the presence of a gas, a pathognomonic finding of a gas-producing infection. Computed tomography also demonstrates any extension of the infection into the surrounding tissue.[50] Some investigators have suggested that CT may be more sensitive than US in the evaluation of patients with severe renal and perirenal infections.[30]

Fine-needle aspiration of a renal abscess helps to determine the infecting organism and the appropriate therapy by Gram stain and culture and antibiotic sensitivities.[41] Thereafter, treatment planning depends on the size, location and number of abscesses, predisposing factors, functional status of the infected kidney, and the general condition of the patient. If the patient is not a surgical candidate, aspiration can be both diagnostic and therapeutic (Fig 7–11). Alternatively, a drainage catheter can be placed within the abscess.[14, 41]

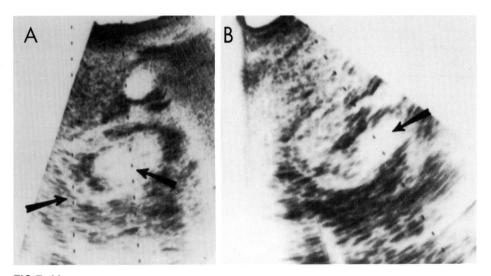

FIG 7–11.
A, supine transverse sonogram demonstrates a renal abscess. Note the internal echoes *(arrow).* **B,** same patient after four weeks of treatment by aspiration and antibiotic therapy. Abscess is smaller in size *(arrow).*

Technique

Selection of the puncture site for abscess aspiration and drainage is made with fluoroscopy, US, or CT. The shortest tract to the abscess is usually chosen; however, to avoid puncture of vital structures, a longer route may be necessary. Entrance into an abscess in the upper renal pole is slightly oblique to avoid entering the lung. The posterior axillary line appears to be a safe landmark to use to avoid entering the peritoneal cavity or colon. The puncture is made in suspended quiet respiration. Initial puncture can be made with a 22-gauge needle. A larger needle may be needed to aspirate thick abscess contents and as much material should be aspirated as is possible.

If placement of a drainage catheter is desired, it can be done at this point, following puncture with an 18-gauge needle, using the standard Seldinger technique. Alternatively, a single stick technique, using a fine-needle and small caliber guidewire, can also be used.

Follow-up evaluation by IV pyelography, US, or CT is necessary to reevaluate abscess size and contour. However, persistence of the mass does not indicate a treatment failure, since it may take months for the cyst to resolve completely.

SOLID RENAL MASSES

Fine-needle aspiration of solid renal masses is rarely indicated, as these masses are typically evaluated and treated surgically. Fine-needle aspiration can be helpful in determining the nature of a primary neoplasm in a nonsurgical candidate and of a renal mass in a patient with another known primary tumor (Fig 7–12).

Fine-Needle Aspiration of Solid Renal Masses

The renal mass is localized by fluoroscopy, US, or CT. Fine-needle aspiration is performed with the needle inserted to a predetermined depth. Wet or dry aspiration biopsy can be performed. Documentation of needle tip position in a solid mass in the kidney (Fig 7–13) or renal bed is sometimes easier with CT (Fig 7–14) than with US. Injection of 1 to 2 ml of air through the biopsy needle can facilitate US visualization (Fig 7–15).

Complications

There are few complications related to fine-needle aspiration of solid renal masses. Von Schreeb and associates[67, 68] followed up a group of patients with renal carcinoma for more than five years. Half of these patients underwent preoperative aspiration biopsy and they showed no evidence of tumor spread along the needle tract or decreased survival.

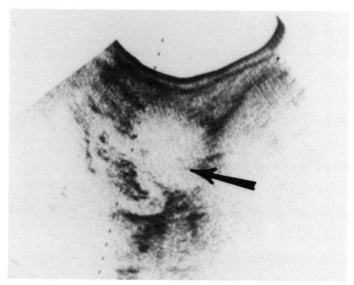

FIG 7–12.
Prone longitudinal sonogram of solid mass *(arrow)* in patient with primary lung malignancy. This mass was a second primary neoplasm, a hypernephroma.

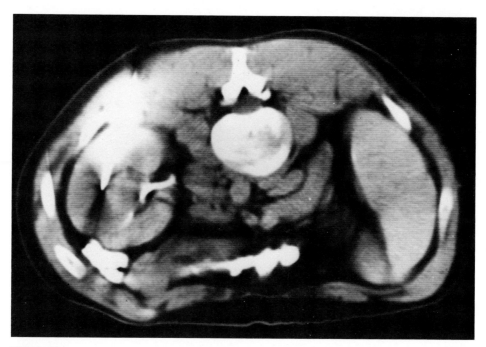

FIG 7–13.
Prone computed tomographic scan taken after the positioning of a 14-gauge Tru-cut needle within a lymphomatous lesion in a patient with a solitary left kidney.

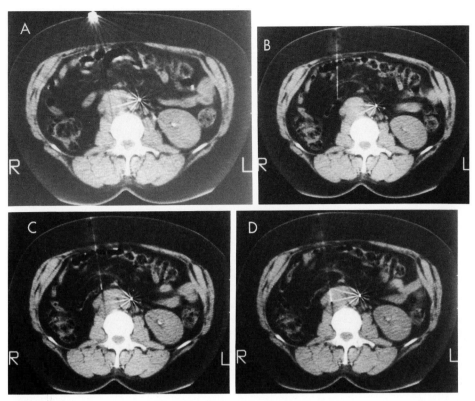

FIG 7–14.
Aspiration biopsy of pericaval nodes in a patient with primary hypernephroma and previous right nephrectomy. **A,** localization; **B,** initial insertion of the 22-gauge needle is too lateral; **C,** redirection of the needle toward the mass; **D,** further advancement of the needle into the mass.

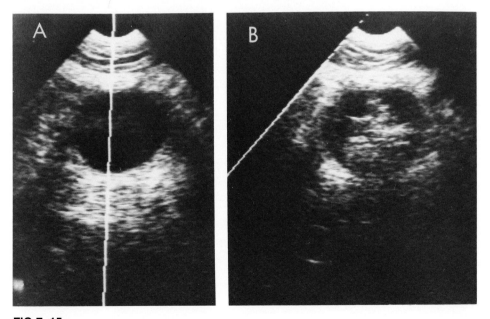

FIG 7–15.
A, mass before cyst puncture. **B,** following fine-needle aspiration, 1 cc of air was injected; note strong echoes produced in center of mass.

RENAL BIOPSY FOR PARENCHYMAL DISEASE

Localization

The value of renal biopsy as a diagnostic procedure in the setting of diffuse parenchymal disease is well recognized. The insignificant morbidity that has been associated with this procedure, as well as the relatively high rate of recovery of renal tissue, is related to the method of localization.[72] Since Iversen and Brun[33] first demonstrated that percutaneous kidney biopsy can be performed without serious complication, techniques of localization have significantly improved.[5] Localization may be accomplished by fluoroscopy with or without IV contrast, radionuclide imaging, US, or CT.

Ultrasonography is the preferred means of localization in most cases. It can be used at the bedside, if necessary. The depth and angle of approach can be accurately determined and the needle tip can be monitored during entry. Hydronephrosis can be detected prior to biopsy with US and follow-up studies can be obtained easily in case of complications.[18, 39] Computed tomography localization is also very valuable, but CT does not provide for continuous visualization of the biopsy needle during placement.

Technique

Usually the right kidney is chosen for biopsy because it is the more caudal in location, making access below the 12th rib easier.[39, 40] The long axis of the kidney is localized with the patient in the prone position. The long axis of the kidney can be easily obtained by real-time sonography. It must be recognized, however, that in the setting of chronic parenchymal disease the kidney may be difficult to visualize. Other technical limitations with US in a particular patient may necessitate the use of CT for localization.

The lower pole of the kidney lateral and inferior to the calyces is the ideal place for biopsy (Fig 7–16). The needle should enter perpendicularly to the posterior surface of the kidney so that it will not deflect into the perinephric space. Localization must be done during suspended respiration, preferably in mid-inspiration to avoid significant movement and dislodgement of the needle after its insertion and to prevent laceration of the kidney. After the proper

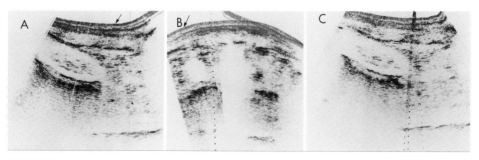

FIG 7–16.
A, prone longitudinal sonography of left kidney; *arrow* shows site of needle puncture. **B,** prone transverse sonography of left kidney. During inspiration, the lower pole is localized *(arrow* shows the intended puncture site). **C,** prone longitudinal sonogram shows angle and depth of approach for kidney biopsy.

angle of approach has been established, the depth from the site of entry to the renal capsule is determined.

To obtain a suitable biopsy specimen for pathologic examination, a tissue core is needed. This necessitates the use of a specially designed renal biopsy needle or a cutting-biopsy needle, such as a Tru-Cut. These needles can be placed under direct visualization with fluoroscopy or US, or in a tandem-approach with a 22-gauge needle. The latter technique would be used more frequently with CT localization. Confirmation of the presence of a sufficient number of glomeruli in the specimen is documented microscopically before the patient is released.

Complications

The primary factors influencing the complication rate of renal biopsy are the size and type of needle and the number of attempts. Accurate localization decreases the number of attempts required to obtain an adequate biopsy and this, coupled with use of a smaller caliber biopsy needle, will decrease the incidence of serious complications such as hematuria, arteriovenous fistulae, and false aneurysms.

Other complications such as subcapsular hematoma (Fig 7–17), retroperitoneal hematoma or urinoma can also be evaluated by US or CT. Vascular complications can be evaluated by dynamic CT, but frequently digital subtraction or conventional angiography is required for diagnosis. Some reported complications, such as pneumothorax, gallbladder perforation, liver or spleen laceration or puncture of the adrenal gland, pancreas, or bowel, should be avoided with more accurate means of localization.[16, 24]

ADRENAL BIOPSY

Technological developments in the imaging modalities of US and CT have resulted in a marked improvement in the radiologic evaluation of the adrenal

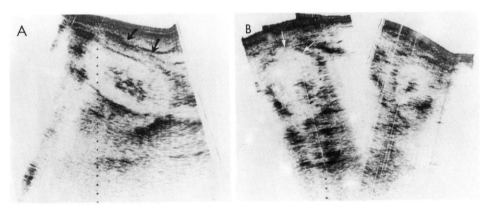

FIG 7–17.
Prone sonogram shows a subcapsular hematoma along the posterior aspect of lower pole of the left kidney following kidney biopsy *(arrows).* Views are **(A)** longitudinal and **(B)** transverse.

glands.[1] Although normal sized adrenals are not easily seen on US examination, they are routinely visualized on CT. Abnormalities of the adrenal gland in patients with evidence of hypersecretion do not typically require preoperative biopsy evaluation. Adrenal masses seen, however, in the context of an asymptomatic patient or a patient with a known malignancy may require percutaneous biopsy for diagnosis. There is a high incidence of benign, nonfunctioning adrenal nodules as determined by autopsy series; therefore the presence of an adrenal mass in a patient with a known or suspected malignancy does not definitely implicate a metastatic lesion.[2, 13]

Nonetheless, metastatic lesions to the adrenal gland are seen in carcinoma of the breast, lung, and stomach, as well as in malignant melanoma. The radiographic appearance of these metastases is nonspecific and the etiology must be determined pathologically. Even normal appearing glands on CT can harbor metastatic disease as shown by percutaneous biopsy.[52]

Percutaneous biopsy of adrenal masses can be accomplished with US[49] or CT guidance.[8, 28] Ultrasonographic guidance may be more difficult to use than CT guidance because of the posterior location of the target lesions and the consequent problems with intercostal approaches. A transhepatic approach to biopsy of the right adrenal can be used with US. Computed tomographic localization of a target lesion in the adrenal gland is probably preferable, as it allows greater flexibility in planning the intended needle course.[56] It is disadvantaged by its inability to precisely define the position of the diaphragm and to follow the needle course during placement.

As with other types of percutaneous biopsy, the diagnostic yield and accuracy of percutaneous adrenal biopsy is high. The diagnostic yield is cited between 90% to 100% for primary and metastatic neoplasms.[8, 28] A low complication rate is reported for these biopsies.[8, 28, 52]

PERINEPHRIC FLUID COLLECTION

Perinephric fluid collections of many different etiologies, including abscess, hematoma, urinoma, and lymphocele, can be characterized and localized by US (Fig 7–18) and CT.[23, 46] Because of the limited ability of these modalities to precisely characterize fluid collections, percutaneous aspiration is useful in the diagnostic evaluation of the fluid collections in the perinephric region. It also provides a route for therapeutic drainage if this is desired.

Perinephric abscesses can occur independently or in association with renal abscesses. In the majority of patients, the abscess is located in the posterior perinephric space. A typical perinephric abscess will contain some internal echoes and have an irregular wall. After the presence of the abscess is confirmed with laboratory findings from fine-needle percutaneous aspiration, the therapeutic course must be determined, i.e., surgical or percutaneous drainage (Fig 7–19). The major indication for surgical treatment is that of a severely diseased or nonfunctioning kidney in association with a perinephric abscess; surgery, in this setting, often follows temporizing management with percutaneous drainage. Thus, percutaneous drainage is often the method of choice of treatment of perinephric abscesses and has proven to be highly efficacious.[23]

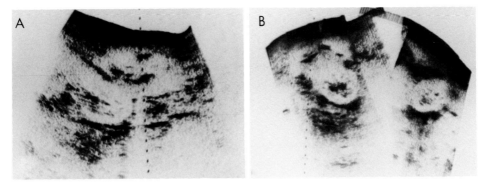

FIG 7–18.
A, prone longitudinal sonogram shows a mass with internal echoes posterior to the kidney. Note strong echoes in the mass, which represent gas bubbles. **B,** prone transverse sonogram of same patient.

However, causes for failure of percutaneous drainage of perinephric abscesses include: (1) inadequate drainage because of small tube size, which can be resolved by simply using a larger catheter; (2) the presence of several pockets of pus, which can be managed by multiple catheter insertions or by separate needle aspirations; and (3) continuous drainage despite acceptable catheter position (Fig 7–20).

Perinephric hematomas can be difficult to aspirate and drain because of their frequently multiloculated and fibrinous nature. Nonetheless, if the patient is symptomatic and not a good surgical candidate, a trial of percutaneous drainage can be attempted. This is especially true for patients who have undergone recent retroperitoneal surgery or who are on anticoagulant therapy. The sonographic appearance of a perinephric hematoma depends on its stage

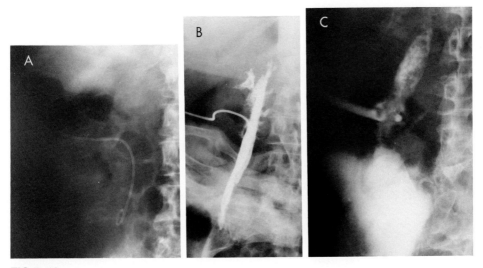

FIG 7–19.
Percutaneous drainage of perinephric abscess by various catheters. **A,** 8.3-F Ring catheter. **B,** 12-F Silastic tube. **C,** large-caliber Foley catheter.

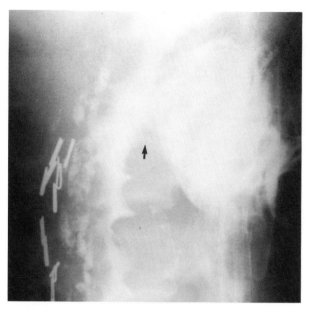

FIG 7–20.
Barium enema demonstrates communication of the colon with perinephric abscess *(arrow)*. The fistula resulted in failure of percutaneous drainage of the abscess.

of development. In the early phase it appears cystic, whereas later with organization it appears more solid and even later, with liquefaction, it appears cystic again. An early hematoma will have a high attenuation coefficient on CT, distinguishing it from other fluid collections.

A urinoma is a collection of extravasated urine that occurs secondary to surgical complications, acute or chronic obstruction, trauma or erosion by calculus, tumor, or inflammatory lesion.[35, 71] If extravasation continues it may be detected by IV urography or radionuclide renogram. Typically, the sonographic appearance is that of a purely cystic mass with posterior acoustic enhancement. Computed tomography may detect very small amounts of extravasated contrast in a urinoma. Percutaneous aspiration can aid in the diagnosis of urinoma when other imaging modalities are nondiagnostic and also provide a means of decompression of the urinoma by simple aspiration or catheter drainage. Treatment of a urinoma, if necessary, depends on the etiological process. In general, decompression of the upper renal collecting system by percutaneous drainage will allow healing of the leak.

A lymphocele is a collection of lymph that may accumulate where lymphatic vessels have been interrupted. This is most commonly seen following retroperitoneal lymph node dissection, radical pelvic surgery and renal transplantation.[21, 34] Following renal transplantation, the frequency of lymphocele has been reported variably from 1% to 15%.[7, 61] Lymphatic leakage can occur from the transplanted kidney or from the recipient lymphatics in the iliac and hypogastric distribution.[11, 21, 26] The incidence of lymphocele formation is directly related to the number of lymph nodes excised.[17] The most frequent symptoms are fullness and pain. The symptoms do not usually become evident until the immediate postoperative discomfort has subsided. If sufficiently large, it may compromise the function of adjacent organs.

Ultrasonography is a sensitive modality for detection of lymphoceles, but it cannot definitely distinguish these from other fluid collections, such as hematoma, abscess, urinoma, or even occasionally, from fluid-filled loops of bowel (Fig 7–21). The CT appearance of lymphocele is also nonspecific, but this modality provides information on the anatomic relationships of the fluid collection to other structures.

Diagnostic and Therapeutic Aspiration of Perinephric Fluid Collections

Localization of perinephric fluid collections is best done with US and CT guidance, though fluoroscopic guidance can be used in selected cases. Simple aspiration or catheter drainage is facilitated by the use of fluoroscopy despite the method of fluid localization. Both fluoroscopy and US allow continuous monitoring of the procedure, whereas CT does not.

After a diagnosis of abscess, hematoma, urinoma, or lymphocele has been established by fine-needle aspiration, a decision must be made as to whether or not further therapeutic measures are needed. Therapeutic options include needle or catheter drainage of the fluid collection.[41, 70] Needle aspiration is used for well-localized, nonseptated, nonviscous fluid collections or urinomas, or some lymphoceles. In these cases the use of sheathed needles with multiple sideholes is preferred for the aspiration. In large or complex urinomas or lymphoceles, or in hematomas and abscesses the placement of a drainage catheter by standard Seldinger techniques is indicated.

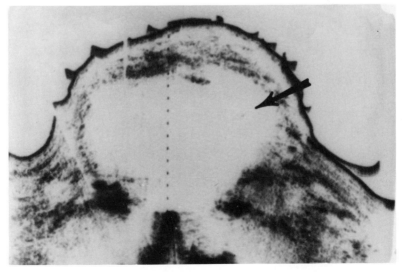

FIG 7–21.
Supine transverse sonogram shows the presence of large fluid collection (lymphocele) *(arrow)* after pelvic lymphadenectomy.

SUMMARY

Percutaneous biopsy of focal renal lesions or of the renal parenchyma in diffuse disease is a safe, reliable, and accurate procedure if performed with precise localization. Ultrasonography and CT provide the best means of localization. Percutaneous drainage, either by simple aspiration or by catheter placement, is an effective means of treatment for many perinephric fluid collections. This is best accomplished with guidance by US, often in conjunction with fluoroscopy, or CT.

REFERENCES

1. Abrams HL, et al: Computed tomography vs. ultrasound of the adrenal gland: A prospective study. *Radiology* 1982; 143:121–128.
2. Abrams JL, Spiro R, Goldstein N: Metastases in carcinoma: Analysis of 1000 autopsied cases. *J Urol* 1959; 81:711–719.
3. Babka JC, Cohen MS, Sode J: Solitary intrarenal cysts causing hypertension. *N Engl J Med* 1974; 291:343–344.
4. Balfe DM, et al: Evaluation of renal masses considered indeterminate on computed tomography. *Radiology* 1982; 142:421–428.
5. Bartels ED, Jorgensen HE: Experiences with percutaneous renal biopsy. *Scand J Urol Nephrol (suppl)* 1972; 15:57.
6. Bean WJ: Renal cyst: Treatment with alcohol. *Radiology* 1981; 138:329–331.
7. Bear RA, et al: Perirenal lymphocyst formation in renal transplant recipients. *Urology* 1976; 7:581.
8. Bernardino ME, et al: CT-guided adrenal biopsy: accuracy, safety and indications. *AJR* 1985; 144:67–69.
9. Caldamone AA, Frank IN: Percutaneous aspiration in the treatment of renal abscess. *J Urol* 1980; 123:92–93.
10. Carson PL, Oughton TV: A model study for diagnosis of small anechoic masses with ultrasound. *Radiology* 1977; 122:765–771.
11. Catalona WJ, Kadmon D, Crane DB: Effect of mini-dose heparin on lymphocele formation following extraperitoneal pelvic lymphadenectomy. *J Urol* 1980; 123:890–892.
12. Coleman BG, et al: Hyperdense renal masses: A computed tomographic dilemma. *AJR* 1984; 143:291–294.
13. Commons RR, Calloway CP: Adenomas of the adrenal cortex. *Arch Intern Med* 1948; 81:37–41.
14. Cronan JJ, Amis ES, Dorfman GS: Percutaneous drainage of renal abscess. *AJR* 1984; 142:351–354.
15. Dean AL: Treatment of solitary cyst of kidney by aspiration. *Trans Am Assoc Genitourin Surg* 1939; 32:91–95.
16. DeBeukelaer MM, et al: Intrarenal arteriovenous fistulas following needle biopsy of the kidney. *J Pediatr* 1971; 78:266–272.
17. Dodd GD, Rutledge F, Wallace S: Postoperative pelvic lymphocysts. *AJR* 1970; 108:312–323.
18. Editorial: Ultrasonically guided renal biopsy. *Arch Intern Med* 1978; 138:355–356.
19. Evans JA, Myers MA, Bosniak MA: Acute renal and perirenal infections. *Semin Roentgenol* 1971; 5:274–291.

20. Fish GW: Large solitary serous cysts of kidney: Report of 32 cases including 2 cases cured by aspiration and instillation of 50% dextrose solution. *JAMA* 1939; 112:514–517.

21. Fried AM, Williams CB, Litvak AS: High retroperitoneal lymphocele: Unusual clinical presentation and diagnosis by ultrasonography. *J Urol* 1980; 123:583–584.

22. Gelman ML, Stone LB: Renal carbuncle: Early diagnosis by retroperitoneal ultrasound. *Urology* 1980; 123:583–584.

23. Gerzof SG, Gale ME: Computed tomography and ultrasonography for diagnosis and treatment of renal and retroperitoneal abscesses. *Urol Clin North Am* 1982; 9:185–193.

24. Giangiacomo J: Inguinal and scrotal ecchymosis as a complication of renal biopsy. *J Urol* 1977; 118:319.

25. Goldman SM, et al: Renal carbuncle: The use of ultrasound in its diagnosis and treatment. *J Urol* 1977; 118:525–527.

26. Gomes AS, et al: Lymphangiography and ultrasound in management of lymphoceles. *Urology* 1979; 13:104–108.

27. Grabstald H: Catheterization of renal cyst for diagnostic and therapeutic purposes. *J Urol* 1954; 71:28–31.

28. Heaston DK, et al: Narrow gauge needle aspiration of solid adrenal masses. *AJR* 1982; 138:1143–1148.

29. Hinman F: Obstructive renal cysts. *J Urol* 1978; 119:681–683.

30. Hoddick W, et al: CT and sonography of severe renal and perirenal infections. *AJR* 1983; 140:517–520.

31. Hotchkiss RS: Perinephric abscess. *Am J Surg* 1953; 85:471–485.

32. Howland WJ, Curry JL: Experimental studies of Pantopaque arachnoiditis: I. Animal studies. *Radiology* 1966; 87:253–261.

33. Iversen P, Brun C: Aspiration biopsy of the kidney. *Am J Med* 1951; 11:324.

34. Kay R, Ruchs E, Barry JM: Management of postoperative pelvic lymphoceles. *Urology* 1980; 15:345–347.

35. Khan AU, Malek RS: Spontaneous urinary extravasation. *J Urol* 1976; 116:161–165.

36. Khashu BL, Seery WH, Rothfeld SH: Nonstaphylococcal bacteria in renal cortical abscess. *Urology* 1976; 7:256–259.

37. Klein DL, Filpi RG: Acute renal carbuncle. *J Urol* 1977; 118:912–918.

38. Koplan JA, et al: Erythropoietin producing renal cyst and polycythemia vera. *Am J Med* 1973; 54:819–824.

39. Kristensen JK: Ultrasonically guided renal biopsy, in: Holm HH, Kristensen JK (eds): *Ultrasonically Guided Puncture Technique.* Philadelphia, WB Saunders Co, 1980, pp 53–54.

40. Kristensen JK, Bartels E, Jorgensen HE: Percutaneous renal biopsy under the guidance of ultrasound. *Scand J Urol Nephrol* 1974; 8:223–226.

41. Kuligowska E, et al: Interventional ultrasound in detection and treatment of renal inflammatory disease. *Radiology* 1983; 147:521–526.

42. Lalli AF: Argument for renal cyst aspiration. *Urology* 1973; 1:523–527.

43. Lang EK: Renal cyst puncture and aspiration: A survey of complications. *AJR* 1977; 128:723–727.

44. Leopold FG, et al: Renal ultrasonography: An updated approach to the diagnosis of renal cysts. *Radiology* 1974; 109:671.

45. Mathe CP: Cystic disease of the kidney: Diagnosis and treatment. *J Urol* 1949; 16:319–326.

46. Mendez G, Isikoff MB, Morillo G: The role of computed tomography in the diagnosis of renal and perirenal abscesses. *J Urol* 1979; 122:582–586.
47. Mindell HJ: Percutaneous renal cyst puncture: Unusual results in two cases. *J Urol* 1975; 114:332–334.
48. Mindell HJ: On the use of Pantopaque in renal cysts. *Radiology* 1976; 119:747–748.
49. Montali G, et al: Sonographically guided fine-needle aspiration biopsy of adrenal masses. *AJR* 1984; 143:1081–1084.
50. Morehouse HT, Weiner SN, Hoffman JC: Imaging in inflammatory disease of the kidney. *AJR* 1984; 143:135–141.
51. Notley RG: Calyceal obstruction due to parapelvic cyst. *Proc R Soc Med* 1971; 64:66.
52. Pagani JJ: Normal adrenal glands in small cell lung carcinoma: CT-guided biopsy. *AJR* 1983; 140:949–951.
53. Peacher WG, Robertson RCL: Absorption of Pantopaque following myelography. *Radiology* 1946; 47:186–187.
54. Pearman RO: Percutaneous needle puncture and aspiration of renal cysts: A diagnostic and therapeutic procedure. *J Urol* 1966; 96:139–145.
55. Pollack HW, et al: The accuracy of gray-scale renal ultrasonography in differentiating cystic neoplasms from benign cysts. *Radiology* 1982; 143:741–745.
56. Price RB, et al: Biopsy of the right adrenal gland by the transhepatic approach. *Radiology* 1983; 148:566.
57. Raskin MD, et al: Percutaneous management of renal cysts: Results of a four-year study. *Radiology* 1975; 115:551–553.
58. Raskin MD, Roen SA, Viamonte M: Effect of intracystic Pantopaque on renal cysts. *J Urol* 1971; 43:646–647.
59. Ross MM, Halpern M, Morrow MW: Evaluation of triple-contrast cyst aspiration in the management of renal masses. *J Urol* 1973; 110:490–493.
60. Sagel SS, et al: Computed tomography of the kidney. *Radiology* 1977; 124:359–370.
61. Starzl TE, et al: Urological complications in 216 human recipients of renal transplants. *Ann Surg* 1970; 172:1.
62. Stevenson JJ, Sherwood T: Conservative management of renal masses. *Br J Urol* 1971; 43:646–647.
63. Thornbury JR: Needle aspiration of avascular renal lesions. *Radiology* 1972; 105:299–302.
64. Truesdale BH, Rous SH, Nelson RP: Perinephric abscess: A review of 26 cases. *J Urol* 1977; 118:910–911.
65. Vestby GW: Percutaneous needle-puncture of renal cysts. New method in therapeutic management. *Invest Radiol* 1967; 2:449–462.
66. Viamonte M, et al: Why every renal mass is not always a surgical lesion: The need for an orderly, logical, diagnostic approach. *J Urol* 1975; 114:190–197.
67. Von Schreeb T, et al: Renal adenocarcinoma: Is there a risk of spreading tumor cells in diagnostic puncture? *Scand J Urol Nephrol* 1967; 1:270–276.
68. Von Schreeb T, Franzen S, Ljungqvist A: Renal adenocarcinoma: Evaluation of malignancy on a cytologic basis: A comparative cytologic and histologic study. *Scand J Urol Nephrol* 1967; 1:265–269.
69. Wahlquist L, Grumstedt B: Therapeutic effect of percutaneous puncture of simple renal cysts: Follow-up investigation of 50 patients. *Acta Clin Scand* 1966; 132:340–347.
70. White M, et al: Percutaneous drainage of post-operative abdominal and pelvic lymphocoeles. *AJR* 1985; 145:1065–1069.

71. Yeh EL, Chang LC, Meade RC: Ultrasound and radionuclide studies of urinary extravasation with hydronephrosis. *J Urol* 1981; 125:728–730.
72. Zeis PM, et al: Ultrasound localization for percutaneous renal biopsy in children. *J Pediatr* 1976; 89:263–268.
73. Zirinsky R, et al: CT of the hyperdense renal cyst: Sonographic correlation. *AJR* 1984; 143:151–156.

Percutaneous Aspiration and Drainage of the Liver Guided by Ultrasound and Computed Tomography

Janis G. Letourneau, M.D.
Morteza K. Elyaderani, M.D.

PERCUTANEOUS BIOPSY OF THE LIVER

Indications for percutaneous liver biopsy include diffuse parenchymal disease or focal hepatic abnormalities that can be solitary or multiple in nature. Liver biopsy as described by Menghini is an accurate means of obtaining diagnostic pathologic material in diffuse hepatic disease.[7, 37] It, however, is not a guided procedure and its diagnostic yield is substantially reduced in the setting of focal hepatic pathology, specifically malignancy (Fig 8–1). Biopsy specimens contain tumor material in 20% to 91% of metastases when obtained by a "blind" technique.[7, 20, 22, 38, 46] Factors that can compromise the diagnostic yield of a "blind" liver biopsy include a small liver size, a deep location of the lesion, and the presence of ascites.

Liver biopsy performed without guided needle placement increases the risk of inadvertent puncture of vascular structures, the biliary tract, and adjacent organs. Ultrasound (US) and computed tomography (CT) can be used to guide percutaneous biopsy in diffuse hepatic disease or in the setting of focal hepatic pathology. Ultrasonographic localization for biopsy, unlike CT localization,

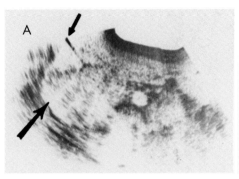 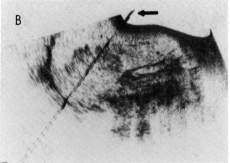

FIG 8–1.
A, supine right anterior sonogram of the liver shows blind biopsy needle tract *(short arrow)* in normal tissue. The mass *(large arrow)* was missed. **B,** supine longitudinal sonogram shows an approach planned for biopsy with a 22-gauge needle in another patient *(arrow).*

provides a means for continuous needle visualization, a factor that may substantially shorten the length of the procedure and thereby further reduce its risks.

Biopsy in Diffuse Parenchymal Disease

When percutaneous biopsy of the liver is done for diagnosis of diffuse parenchymal disease, placing the patient in a supine oblique decubitus position with the right side up will facilitate obtaining an adequate specimen because of the posterior location of the liver. Large (16- and 18-gauge) needles with cutting tips are preferred for biopsy in this situation (Fig 8–2). A smaller needle may be used if the risk of bleeding is high.

Biopsy of Focal Hepatic Lesions

Focal hepatic lesions occur as the result of many disease processes. Fine-needle aspiration biopsy is a useful technique to establish or confirm the diagnosis of such a lesion. Localization of the mass within the liver is critical to the success of the procedure and should be performed with US or CT.[3]

Most common focal hepatic lesions include neoplasm, abscess, and cysts. In a cumulative review of 221 patients who underwent percutaneous aspiration biopsy, a diagnostic accuracy of 89% was seen in malignancies and an accuracy of 100% was seen in benign processes such as infection and cysts.[4, 14, 41, 46, 52] The predictive value of negative results was, however, low. The incidence of significant complication with such a biopsy is quite low and was reported in one of 120 aspiration biopsies, and two of 139 cutting biopsies.[36]

The US features of focal hepatic masses are usually either those of a solid or complex mass or those of a cyst. Focal hepatic lesions are typically low attenuation on CT, although high-dense and iso-dense abnormalities are occasionally identified. Both US and CT can be used for localization of a focal liver lesion for percutaneous aspiration biopsy. Real-time sonography offers the advantage of continuous visualization of the biopsy procedure (Fig 8–3).

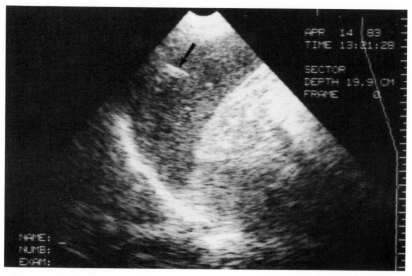

FIG 8–2.
Supine transverse sonogram of the liver with the patient in a right anterior oblique position shows the tip of the Tru-cut needle within the liver parenchyma *(arrow).*

Solid or Complex Masses

Focal hepatic lesions that are solid or complex in nature by US are most likely neoplastic, primary or secondary, and less likely, inflammatory. The sonographic appearances of primary and secondary neoplasms of the liver can be similar, but the pattern of distribution may vary. Primary hepatic tumors, most commonly hepatomas in the adult patient population, are characterized by a complex pattern of echogenicity, with areas of both high and low level echo-intensity, in an often infiltrative pattern. Hepatomas may be solitary or multi-centric.[5, 33, 55] They may also occur in the setting of hepatic cirrhosis, which can be associated with overall increased echogenicity of the liver and loss of detail

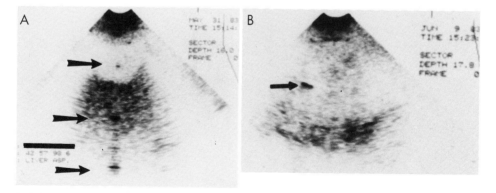

FIG 8–3.
A, sector real-time sonogram of a liver mass shows the needle tip in the central portion of the mass. Note reverberation artifact of needle tip *(arrows.)* **B,** needle tip seen in the periphery of a liver lesion *(arrow)* in a different patient.

in the parenchyma and around the triads.[8] Hepatoblastoma is the most common primary hepatic neoplasm in children. Its sonographic appearance is also that of a solid mass, often with ill-defined margins.[6] Cavernous hemangiomas are the most common benign neoplasms in the liver. These classically are well-circumscribed lesions of variable size, with a high degree of echogenicity, sometimes in association with posterior acoustic enhancement, reflecting their vascular character.[24] Their nature can be confirmed with nuclear[39, 44] or dynamic CT examinations. Secondary liver neoplasms, metastases, can be solitary or multiple. Their sonographic appearances are manifold and can range from poorly to well circumscribed and from hypoechoic to hyperechoic. The degree of sonographic heterogeneity within a hepatic metastasis is variable as well; lesions may have a central hypoechoic core or a surrounding hypoechoic halo.[51] Inflammatory lesions of the liver, most commonly pyogenic or amebic abscesses, are complex lesions by ultrasound, containing a variable cystic component and often some degree of septation.[31, 40, 45, 54]

The CT appearance of neoplastic and inflammatory hepatic disease is nonspecific and reflects their complex pathologic features. Most such lesions are at least in part of low attenuation. Primary neoplasms, most commonly hepatomas and cholangiocarcinomas, are usually of mixed attenuation status.[32, 33] Hepatoblastomas may have calcification readily detected by CT.[29] As mentioned earlier, dynamic CT techniques are of value in diagnosing vascular hepatic neoplasms.[2, 25, 26] Metastases are typically low-dense relative to the liver parenchyma and can have a mixed attenuation pattern.[59] Abscesses are quite variable in their appearance, often with central areas of low attenuation and septations. These may also be multifocal.[48]

Percutaneous aspiration biopsy can be safely performed in all neoplastic and inflammatory lesions of the liver with the possible exceptions of cavernous hemangiomas (because of the risk of hemorrhage with larger needles)[35] and echinococcal cysts (because of the risk of anaphylaxis).[49] The liver is thoroughly evaluated with US or CT and a site is chosen for biopsy. When multiple lesions are present, the lesion chosen will depend on many factors, including its size, location, and relationship to biliary and vascular structures. Computed tomographic localization may be preferred with small and/or deep lesions.

Percutaneous biopsy of liver lesions should be done with the patient in suspended respiration. Many different techniques can be used with US (Fig 8–4) or CT guidance (Fig 8–5), including multiple directed passes, tandem needle punctures, or coaxial aspirations. An angled needle tract may be necessary to avoid thoracic structures. Polyethylene tubing connecting the aspirating needle and the syringe allow flexibility of the system that may be desirable because of the respiratory motion of the liver.

Special mention must be made of biopsy of lesions that obstruct the major bile ducts. These can be primary neoplasms originating from the pancreas, bile ducts, or gallbladder or secondary deposits originating from a variety of primary tumors. Inflammatory processes can also less commonly produce masses in this region. Diagnostic evaluation may be difficult in these cases and percutaneous biopsy of the mass or brush biopsy of the biliary ducts may be valuable for determining patient management. Percutaneous biopsy can be guided by US. It can, however, be facilitated by the injection of contrast in the biliary

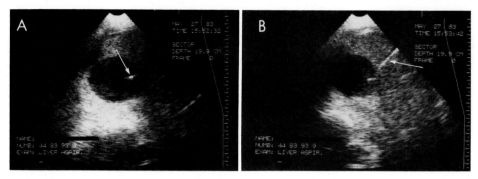

FIG 8–4.
Real-time ultrasonography demonstrates a complex mass, primarily cystic, but with internal echoes. Note tip of needle **(A)** and needle tract **(B)** *(arrow)*.

system to define the extent of the mass and then guided by fluoroscopy or CT. Brush, guidewire, or auger biopsy of such lesions can be performed during or following percutaneous transhepatic cholangiography and placement of a drainage catheter[9, 11] (Figs 8–6, 8–7, and 8–8).

Hepatic Cysts

Benign hepatic cysts that are not parasitic in origin are usually congenital in nature. They can be single or multiple, variable in size, and infrequently

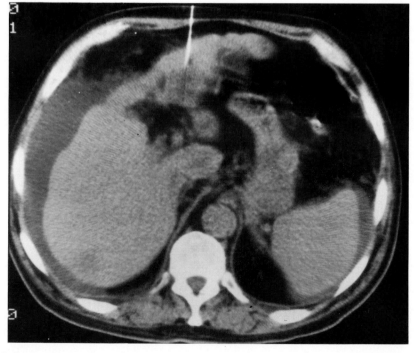

FIG 8–5.
Percutaneous biopsy specimen of a liver metastasis in a patient with an adenocarcinoma of the pancreas. Following fine-needle localization, multiple biopsy specimens were taken using a tandem approach.

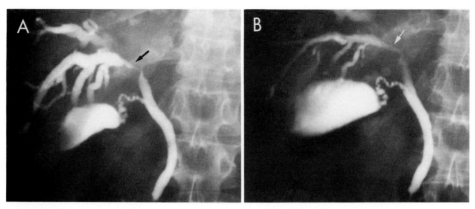

FIG 8–6.
A, transhepatic cholangiogram shows a stricture of distal right hepatic duct *(arrow).* **B,** the catheter is wedged in the proximal extent of the stricture for brush biopsy *(arrow).*

multiloculated. Their fluid contents may be thin or thick and vary in color from clear to yellow. Congenital cysts occur more frequently in females than in males, with a ratio of 4:1. Complications include hemorrhage, infection, and rupture either into the biliary ductal system or into the free peritoneal cavity.

On sonographic examination, hepatic cysts are well-circumscribed sonolucent masses with associated posterior acoustic enhancement (Fig 8–9,A). The features of a simple cyst are also demonstrated on CT, with a hepatic cyst seen as a well-defined area of water or near-water density (Fig 8–9,B). The low at-

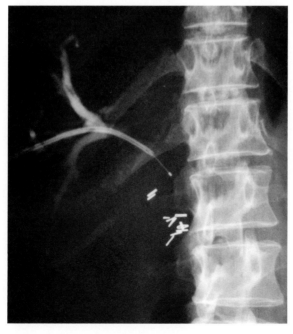

FIG 8–7.
Brush biopsy guidewire in the area of the stricture in the right hepatic duct. (From Elyaderani MK, et al: *Radiology* 1980; 135:777–778. Reproduced by permission.)

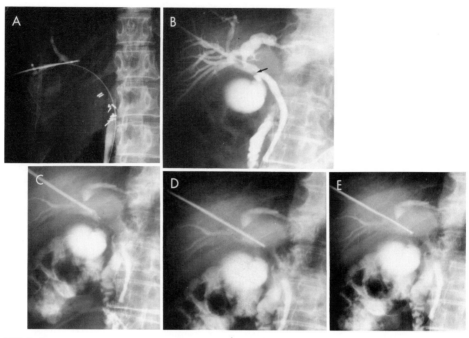

FIG 8–8.
Forceps biopsy of the right hepatic duct. **A,** guidewire is situated within the common duct. (From Elyaderani MK, et al: *Radiology* 1980; 135:777–778. Reproduced by permission.) **B,** cholangiogram shows defect *(arrow)* in proximal common hepatic duct. **C,** 10-F catheter is positioned adjacent to the intraluminal defect (same as that shown in **B**). **D,** Olympus forceps passed through catheter up to the mass. **E,** the cutting edge of forceps is opened and biopsy is performed.

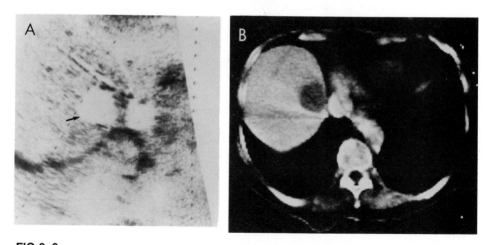

FIG 8–9.
A, transverse sonogram (patient supine) of the liver shows a simple hepatic cyst adjacent to the inferior vena cava *(arrow)*. **B,** computed tomographic scan of same patient shows sharply defined, homogeneous mass with near-water density.

tenuation of small cysts may be difficult to verify because of partial volume averaging. Despite these relatively characteristic features, other diagnostic possibilities exist for such US and CT appearances. These include neoplasm, inflammatory lesions, and biloma (Fig 8–10).[1] The lack of specificity of the CT findings has been well described.[13] Because of this, percutaneous aspiration biopsy can be helpful in differentiating benign hepatic cysts from other cavitary or cystic processes.

Percutaneous aspiration of hepatic cysts detected incidentally by US or CT examination is often not necessary. However, it may be desirable to rule out other diagnostic possibilities, as mentioned earlier. In these instances the procedure can be performed under either US or CT guidance. Alternatively, if the lesion is causing symptoms, because of its size or coexistent infection or hemorrhage, aspiration may sometimes be therapeutic as well as diagnostic.[47, 50] Complicating infection or hemorrhage can also be seen occasionally in patients with inherited polycystic disease of the liver.

Usually, catheter drainage of hepatic cysts is not indicated. Sclerosis of cysts can be accomplished with percutaneous instillation of iophendylate (Pantopaque).[16] However, possible communication with vascular or biliary structures should be ruled out before this is done.

DRAINAGE OF HEPATIC ABSCESSES

Hepatic abscess is a serious illness, but early diagnosis and precise localization of the lesion by US[15] reduce the mortality rate. The US and CT features of

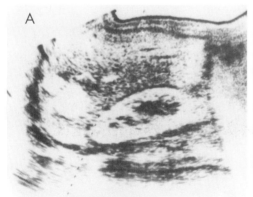
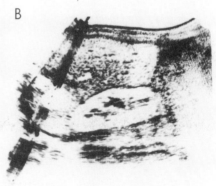
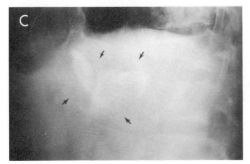

FIG 8–10.
A, supine longitudinal sonogram shows cystic mass in the posterior aspect of liver following trauma. **B,** after localization, the angle of approach is determined. **C,** cystogram *(arrows)* is performed after aspiration of bile.

abscesses are diverse; therefore, to obtain a rapid definitive diagnosis, fine-needle aspiration is recommended.[61] Percutaneous cholangiography[19] and radionuclide scintigraphy[12] are indicated in selected cases.

Most hepatic abscesses are round or oval sonolucent masses with irregularity of the wall.[10, 40] Fine, coarse, and clumpy internal echoes may be seen and occasionally there is a fluid-debris interface in the abscess cavity. The abscesses that contain air may be seen as densely echogenic masses with or without acoustic shadowing.[30] The location of an abscess does not seem to be a significant discriminating factor for sonographic differential diagnosis. Even small abscesses may now be detected by US because of technical improvements in the equipment, resulting in better spatial resolution.

The sonographic appearance of hepatic abscesses can resemble that of necrotic neoplasms,[60] infected cysts, hematomas, traumatic bilomas, simple cysts, and echinococcal cysts (Fig 8–11) and also that of an intrahepatic gallbladder. The accuracy of US in the diagnosis of cystic hepatic lesions, aided by available clinical information, is reported to be 90%.[40]

On CT examination, an abscess is an area of decreased attenuation within the liver. The peripheral rim may be enhanced by contrast medium due to the inflammatory nature of the lesion. The margin of the lesion can be well or poorly circumscribed (Figs 8–12 and 8–13). Septations and loculations within the abscess may be present.[23, 48] Demonstration of gas within the fluid collection increases the likelihood that it is an abscess. Fluid collections other than abscesses can create the same appearance, and the following lesions must be considered in differential diagnosis: chronic hematomas, bilomas, traumatic cysts, neoplasms, and infected cysts.

Adequate drainage remains the cornerstone of treatment of pyogenic or

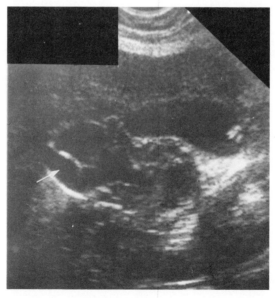

FIG 8–11.
Supine longitudinal sonogram of a hepatic echinococcal cyst; note internal complexity of the lesion *(arrow).*

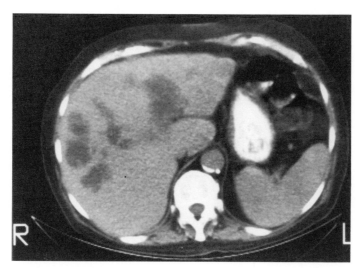

FIG 8–12.
Computed tomographic scan of liver abscess.

amebic hepatic abscesses. Percutaneous catheter drainage of liver abscesses yields excellent results[27, 57] and is applicable to single or multiple lesions when used in conjunction with appropriate antibacterial or antiparasitic medication (Fig 8–14). It has a special applicability in the setting of amebic abscess where open surgical drainage may be complicated by secondary infection or fistula

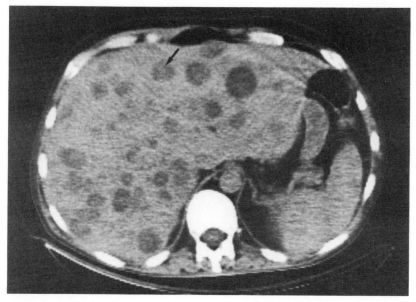

FIG 8–13.
Computed tomographic scan of the liver demonstrates numerous candidal abscesses, some with relatively soft-tissue attenuation values *(arrow).*

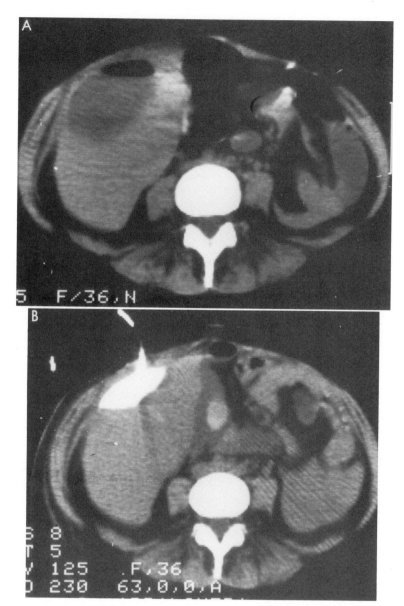

FIG 8–14.
A, computed tomographic scan of a patient with Crohn's disease with a large hepatic abscess demonstrates an air-fluid level. **B,** computed tomographic scan of the same patient following percutaneous catheter drainage of the abscess. Some contrast has been instilled into the abscess cavity. (Courtesy of Jeffrey R. Crass, M.D., Univ. of Minnesota).

formation.[43, 56] Percutaneous aspiration of suspected echinococcal cysts or abscesses should be avoided because of the risk of systemic anaphylaxis.

The site for needle puncture and subsequent drainage is selected under the guidance of US[18] or CT[20, 35] (Fig 8–15,A). Selecting a safe route into the abscess is the most crucial step in percutaneous aspiration. The route should be as short and as direct as possible. The location of structures such as loops of bowel, major vessels, the gallbladder, and the pleural cavity should be determined in relation to percutaneous access. Extension of the pleural cavity around the liver especially limits puncture site selection. The puncture site should avoid the pleural cavity, not only to prevent possible pneumothorax and contamination, but to reduce patient discomfort and to reduce the possibility of sympathetic pleural effusion. Sonography is very useful in localizing the diaphragm and, therefore, the pleural cavity.

Anterolateral, midaxillary, or posterolateral approaches are preferred for catheter drainage. An anterior approach often has limited usefulness because

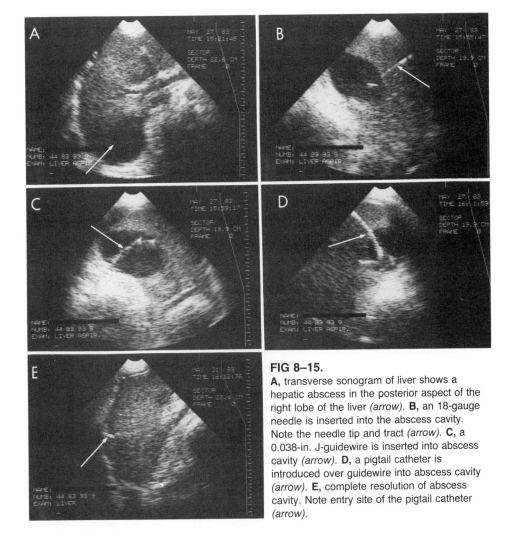

FIG 8–15.
A, transverse sonogram of liver shows a hepatic abscess in the posterior aspect of the right lobe of the liver *(arrow).* **B,** an 18-gauge needle is inserted into the abscess cavity. Note the needle tip and tract *(arrow).* **C,** a 0.038-in. J-guidewire is inserted into abscess cavity *(arrow).* **D,** a pigtail catheter is introduced over guidewire into abscess cavity *(arrow).* **E,** complete resolution of abscess cavity. Note entry site of the pigtail catheter *(arrow).*

of the intervening gallbladder and loops of bowel, and a posterior approach is usually not comfortable for the patient.

Initial aspiration of the abscess can be done with a fine needle. Catheter drainage can then be performed using a single-stick technique with an 0.018-in. guidewire system or a tandem needle approach using a larger gauge needle and the Seldinger technique or a needle-sheath system like that used for translumbar aortography (Fig 8–15,B, C, and D). Ideally, catheter manipulation is performed with fluoroscopic guidance. The catheter must be placed with all of its sideholes within the abscess cavity to tamponade the hepatic vessels and to limit leakage around the catheter.

An 8.3-French (F) catheter is adequate to drain many hepatic abscesses (Fig 8–15,E), although those that contain large amounts of debris and necrotic material may fail to drain even with larger catheters. Multiple abscess cavities without communications must be drained by multiple catheters[17, 34, 42] (Fig 8–16).

Irrigation of the abscess cavity with normal saline is valuable in that it prevents catheter blockage and also loosens the necrotic material for better drainage. Triluminal sump catheters can be used to irrigate continuously, at low pressures. When irrigating through standard catheters, irrigation must be gentle and the volume of saline should not exceed the volume of the abscess cavity. Vigorous irrigation may produce contamination and sepsis.

A review of 52 cases in the literature reveals an overall rate of success of 82% in percutaneous hepatic abscess drainage.[14, 41, 42, 53, 58] Reasons for failed percutaneous drainage included: (1) premature removal of the drainage catheter, (2) placement of drainage catheter in infected or necrotic tumors, (3) presence of associated bile leak, and (4) presence of multiloculated cavity or diffusely phlegmonous liver.

Therefore, percutaneous drainage of hepatic abscesses is a well-tolerated and generally successful procedure. The probability of favorable outcome is reduced by the presence of a multiloculated fluid collection or associated bile leak, as seen following trauma. These unfavorable factors can be reduced by placement of multiple drainage catheters and by percutaneous biliary diversion, respectively.

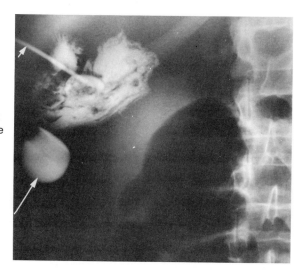

FIG 8–16.
Large Foley catheter *(large arrow)* and 8.3-F pigtail catheter *(short arrow)* positioned within two adjacent hepatic abscesses. The balloon of the catheter is distended by diluted contrast material. Minimal contrast material was injected through the pigtail catheter to demonstrate the extent of the abscess cavity.

ASPIRATION AND DRAINAGE OF PERIHEPATIC FLUID COLLECTIONS

Perihepatic fluid collections, generally located in the subphrenic, subhepatic, and subcapsular spaces and in the region of the porta hepatis, are most commonly abscesses, bilomas, hematomas, or localized accumulations of ascites. Ultrasonography and CT are accurate in localizing these collections for diagnostic aspiration and for guiding therapeutic drainage if indicated. The topic of perihepatic abscess is discussed elsewhere in this text and will not be reviewed here.

Bilomas occur as complications of surgery, trauma, or cholangiography, percutaneous or endoscopic.[28] Usually these are located near the main biliary ducts or in the gallbladder fossa. Evacuation of the biloma can be accomplished by catheter drainage, accompanied by percutaneous biliary diversion. If the biliary leak is large and in the extrahepatic portion of the biliary tree, tamponade of the tear by a large catheter may allow the leak to seal off. As with all fluid collections, aspiration can be performed with a fine needle, catheter drainage can be accomplished by a variety of techniques, including a single-stick method or the Seldinger-type catheter placement. Ultrasonographic and CT localization is often aided by fluoroscopy for drainage catheter placement.

Percutaneous fine-needle aspiration can establish the diagnosis of hematoma or loculated ascites in the perihepatic spaces. Occasionally, aspiration of a hematoma will require the use of a larger needle. A fluid collection of this nature does not usually require catheter drainage. However, US- or CT-guided catheter drainage of selected patients with infected perihepatic hematomas or ascites may be indicated.

SUMMARY

Fine-needle percutaneous aspiration under US or CT guidance can be used to establish the diagnosis of hepatic masses and perihepatic fluid collections. Therapeutic catheter drainage of certain hepatic and perihepatic fluid collections can also be accomplished using US or CT localization, with guidewire and catheter manipulation facilitated by fluoroscopy.

Acknowledgement

We thank Jeffrey R. Crass, M.D., for providing the case material for the figure depicting CT localization of an hepatic abscess.

REFERENCES

1. Barnes PA, Thomas JL, Bernardino ME: Pitfalls in the diagnosis of hepatic cysts by computed tomography. *Radiology* 1981; 141:129–133.
2. Barnett PH, et al: Computed tomography in the diagnosis of cavernous hemangioma of the liver. *AJR* 1980; 134:439–447.
3. Bjork RT, Foley WD, Varma RR: Percutaneous liver biopsy in difficult cases simplified by CT or ultrasonic localization. *Dig Dis Sci* 1981; 26:145–158.

4. Bondestam S, et al: Ultrasound-guided fine needle biopsy of mass lesions affecting the hepatobiliary tract. *Acta Radiol (Diagn) (Stockh)* 1981; 22:549–551.

5. Broderick TW, et al: Echographic and radionuclide detection of hepatoma. *Radiology* 1980; 135:149–151.

6. Brunelle F, Chaumont P: Hepatic tumors in children: Ultrasonic differentiation of malignant from benign lesions. *Radiology* 1984; 150:695–699.

7. Conn HO, Yesmer R: A re-evaluation of needle biopsy in diagnosis of metastatic cancer of the liver. *Ann Intern Med* 1963; 59:51–53.

8. Cottone M, et al: Ultrasound in the diagnosis of hepatocellular carcinoma associated with cirrhosis. *Radiology* 1983; 147:517–519.

9. Cropper LD, Gold RE: Simplified brush biopsy of the bile ducts. *Radiology* 1984; 148:307–308.

10. Dodds WJ, Goldberg HL: Hepatic abscess: Ultrasound as an aid to diagnosis. *Forums Gastrointest Roentgenol Digest Dis* 1977; 22:33–37.

11. Elyaderani MK, Gabriele OF: Brush and forceps biopsy of biliary ducts via percutaneous transhepatic catheterization. *Radiology* 1980; 135:777–778.

12. Elyaderani MK, Gabriele OF: Comparison of radionuclide imaging and ultrasonography of the liver. *South Med J* 1983; 76:37–44.

13. Federle MP, Filly RA, Moss AA: Cystic hepatic neoplasms: Complementary roles of CT and sonography. *AJR* 1981; 136:345–348.

14. Ferrucci JT Jr, et al: Diagnosis of abdominal malignancy by radiologic fine-needle aspiration biopsy. *AJR* 1980; 134:323–330.

15. Gerzof SG, et al: Percutaneous catheter drainage of abdominal abscesses guided by ultrasound and computed tomography. *AJR* 1979; 133:1–8.

16. Goldstein HM, Carlyle DR, Nelson RS: Treatment of symptomatic hepatic cyst by percutaneous instillation of Pantopaque. *AJR* 1976; 127:850–853.

17. Greenwood LH, Collins TL, Yrizarry JM: Percutaneous management of multiple liver abscesses. *AJR* 1982; 139:390–392.

18. Gronvall S, et al: Drainage of abdominal abscesses guided by sonography. *AJR* 1982; 138:527–529.

19. Grossman RI, et al: Diagnosis of pyogenic hepatic abscesses by percutaneous transhepatic cholangiography. *AJR* 1979; 132:919–920.

20. Haaga JR, Alfidi RJ: Definitive treatment of a large pyogenic liver abscess with CT guidance. *Clev Clin Q* 1976; 43:85–88.

21. Haaga JR, Alfidi RJ: Precise biopsy localization by computed tomography. *Radiology* 1976; 118:603–607.

22. Haaga JR, Vanek J: Computed tomographic guided liver biopsy using the Menghini needle. *Radiology* 1979; 133:405–408.

23. Halverson RA, et al: The variable CT appearance of hepatic abscesses. *AJR* 1984; 141:941–946.

24. Itai Y, et al: Computed tomography and sonography of cavernous hemangiomas of the liver. *AJR* 1983; 141:315–320.

25. Itai Y, et al: Computed tomography of cavernous hemangioma of the liver. *Radiology* 1980; 137:149–155.

26. Johnson CM, et al: Computed tomography and angiography of cavernous hemangiomas of the liver. *Radiology* 1981; 138:115–121.

27. Johnson RD, et al: Percutaneous drainage of pyogenic liver abscesses. *AJR* 1985; 144:463–467.

28. Juler GL, Conroy RM, Fuelleman RW: Bile leakage following percutaneous transhepatic cholangiography with the Chiba needle. *Arch Surg* 1977; 112:954–958.

29. Korobkin M, et al: Computed tomography of primary liver tumors in children. *Radiology* 1981; 139:431–435.

30. Kressel HY, Filly FA: Ultrasonographic appearance of gas-containing abscesses in the abdomen. *AJR* 1978; 130:71–73.
31. Kuligowska E, Connors SK, Shapiro JH: Liver abscess: Sonography in diagnosis and treatment. *AJR* 1982; 138:253–257.
32. Kunstlinger F, et al: Computed tomography of hepatocellular carcinoma. *AJR* 1980; 134:431–437.
33. LaBerge JM, et al: Hepatocellular carcinoma: Assessment of resectability by computed tomography and ultrasound. *Radiology* 1984; 152:485–490.
34. Martin EC, et al: Percutaneous drainage in the management of hepatic abscesses. *Surg Clin North Am* 1981; 61:157–167.
35. Martino CR, Haaga JR: Percutaneous biopsy of the liver. *Semin Intervent Radiol* 1985; 2:245–253.
36. Martino CR, et al: CT-guided liver biopsies: Eight years' experience. *Radiology* 1984; 152:755–757.
37. Menghini G: One-second needle biopsy of the liver. *Gastroenterology* 1958; 35:190–199.
38. Menghini G: One-second biopsy of the liver: Problems in its clinical application. *N Engl J Med* 1979; 283:582–585.
39. Moinuddin M, et al: Scintigraphic diagnosis of hepatic hemangioma: Its role in the management of hepatic mass lesions. *AJR* 1985; 145:223–228.
40. Newlin N, et al: Ultrasonic features of pyogenic liver abscess. *Radiology* 1981; 139:155–159.
41. Nosher JL, Plafker J: Fine-needle aspiration of the liver with ultrasound guidance. *Radiology* 1980; 136:177–180.
42. Novy SB, et al: Pyogenic liver abscess: Angiographic diagnosis and treatment by closed aspiration. *AJR* 1974; 121:338–395.
43. Patterson HD: Open aspiration for solitary liver abscess. *Am J Surg* 1970; 119:326.
44. Rabinowitz SA, McKusick KA, Strauss HW: [99m]Tc red blood cell scintigraphy in evaluating focal liver lesions. *AJR* 1984; 143:63–68.
45. Ralls PW, et al: Sonographic findings in hepatic amebic abscess. *Radiology* 1982; 145:123–126.
46. Rasmussen SN, et al: Ultrasonically guided liver biopsy. *Br Med J* 1972; 2:5500–5502.
47. Roemer CE, et al: Hepatic cysts: Diagnosis and therapy by sonographic needle aspiration. *AJR* 1981; 136:1065–1070.
48. Rubinson HA, Isikoff MB, Hill MC: Diagnostic imaging of hepatic abscesses: A retrospective analysis. *AJR* 1980; 135:735–740.
49. Saidi F: *Surgery Hydatid Disease.* Philadelphia, WB Saunders Co, 1976.
50. Saini S, et al: Percutaneous aspiration of hepatic cysts does not provide definitive therapy. *AJR* 1983; 141:559–560.
51. Scheible W, Gosink BB, Leopold GR: Gray scale echographic patterns of hepatic metastatic disease. *AJR* 1977; 129:983–987.
52. Schwark WB, Schmite-Moorman P: Ultrasonically guided fine-needle biopsies in neoplastic liver disease: Cytohistologic diagnoses and echo pattern of lesions. *Cancer* 1981; 48:1469–1477.
53. Stephenson RF, Guzzetta LR, Tagulinao OA: CT-guided Seldinger catheter drainage of a hepatic abscess. *AJR* 1978; 131:323–324.
54. Sukov RJ, Cohen LR, Sample WF: Sonography of hepatic amebic abscesses. *AJR* 1980; 134:911–915.
55. Tanaka S, et al: Hepatocellular carcinoma: Sonographic and histologic correlation. *AJR* 1983; 140:701–707.
56. Turrill FL, Burnham JR: Hepatic amebiasis. *Am J Surg* 1966; 111:424.

57. vanSonnenberg E, et al: Intrahepatic amebic abscess: Indications for and results of percutaneous catheter drainage. *Radiology* 1985; 156:631–635.

58. vanSonnenberg E, et al: Percutaneous drainage of abscesses and fluid collections: Technique, results, and applications. *Radiology* 1982; 142:1–10.

59. Wooten WB, Bernardino ME, Goldstein HM: Computed tomography of necrotic hepatic metastases. *AJR* 1978; 131:839–842.

60. Wooten WB, Green B, Goldstein HM: Ultrasonography of necrotic hepatic metastases. *Radiology* 1978; 128:447–450.

61. Zornoza J, et al: Fine-needle aspiration biopsy of the liver. *AJR* 1980; 134:331–334.

9

Percutaneous Drainage of Abscesses

Eric C. Martin, M.A. (Oxon.), M.R.C.P., F.R.C.R.
Karen J. Laffey, M.D., Ph.D.

In 1979 Gerzof and co-workers[4] published a landmark paper that reintroduced the technique of percutaneous drainage of abscesses. The chief author's background was in ultrasound (US) and computed tomography (CT), and it is clear now that the major impetus for percutaneous abscess drainage stemmed from the enormous advantages of cross-sectional imaging, rather than from the expansion of percutaneous interventional techniques. Certainly, abscess drainage has been widely practiced by interventional radiologists, and certainly interventional radiologists were expanding their field enormously at that time, but it would seem that they were not responsible for the development of the procedure, but only for its popularization. Pride of place must go to the cross-sectional imagers, for many of whom abscess drainage, and perhaps percutaneous biopsy, is their only interventional practice. The explanation lies in the enormously increased tissue resolution obtainable with cross-sectional imaging, which makes an abdominal abscess as visible to the radiologist as an empyema.

Empyemas are, of course, drained percutaneously. That this is the case seems natural because an empyema is so distinctly visualized on the chest film where radiolucent lung silhouettes the dense pleural fluid. This fluid, placed as it is just beneath the chest wall a few centimeters from the skin, is a tempting target for percutaneous aspiration. The fact that the technique is performed as a surgical procedure, with a small incision and perhaps a partial rib resection, reflects the habits of the operator rather than the complexity of the approach. Surgical custom alone dictates that drainage is best accomplished through an incision.[14]

Modern US and body CT effectively provide the same visualization of the abdomen that we are accustomed to in the chest, and once one can see an abscess as clearly as one sees an empyema, it is natural to consider draining it percutaneously. Once a puncture is performed, the means of exchanging that needle for a catheter are well established.[21, 32]

The vastly increased tissue resolution of US and CT compared with plain abdominal films and the resultant increase in intra-abdominal visibility allow for much earlier diagnosis of abscesses and for far better localization. It is primarily this improved diagnostic capability that has contributed to the decreased mortality reported in radiologic as opposed to surgical series. That earlier diagnosis leads to a lower mortality is well documented in the surgical literature. In 1979, DeCosse et al.[3] reported a series of 60 subphrenic abscesses with an overall mortality rate of 43%; the rate fell to 25% among those patients in whom adequate drainage (by implication, early drainage) was established.

The literature describing hepatic abscesses best illustrates the situation. In 1948, effectively in the preantibiotic era, Ochsner et al.[22] reported a large series of hepatic abscesses: 47 in their own patients and 518 described in the literature. The overall mortality rate was 79% and the untreated mortality rate was 100%. In 1975, much later and well into the antibiotic era, Pitt and Zuidema[23] reported a series of 80 patients with hepatic abscesses. The overall mortality rate was 65%. A subset of their patients with solitary abscesses who received adequate antibiotics and adequate drainage had a mortality rate of only 8%.

Yet, despite the influence of this subset of 24 patients, the overall mortality figures remained essentially unchanged from the series reported in 1948. Pitt and Zuidema[23] noted that 20% of the patients died within 24 hours of admission. The implication is not that antibiotics make only a small contribution to the management of abscesses, but rather that hepatic abscesses continued to be missed, or diagnosed late, even up to 1975. Such a state of affairs should not exist today with the imaging advantages of US and CT. The legitimate mortality rate for hepatic abscesses should remain in single figures.

HISTORY

For centuries, pointing abscesses have been treated percutaneously with wide incision and open drainage, and both Celsus and Hippocrates described the use of intra-abdominal cannulas to evacuate abdominal collections. Yates[36] recounted much of the early history of abscess drainage in an elegant monograph. The triad of wide incision under direct vision, disruption of loculations, and dependent drainage with large-bore catheters has become the sine qua non of surgical management.

In the Lettsomian lectures to the Royal College of Surgeons, London, Rogers[28] presented his results on the use of repeated aspiration of amebic liver abscesses using a 14-gauge needle. Although repeated aspiration reduced the mortality rate from 68% to 14%, Rogers' report fell on apparently stony ground. Thirty years later, McFadzean et al.[19] reported successful percutaneous drainage of 14 hepatic abscesses, again using a 14-gauge needle with an average of three punctures per abscess. Of particular note is that the diagnosis was made and drainage instituted in all these patients within 24 hours of their admission to hospital. All 14 were cured and none had recurrence. Again the report was ignored.

It was not until 1979 that Gerzof and associates reintroduced the procedure with a report of 24 patients, and by 1981 they had expanded the series to 67 patients.[5] In 1982, we reported the drainage in 42 patients,[12] and van Sonnenberg reported on drainage in 51 patients.[33] The overall mortality rate reported in these series is in single figures, with cure rates of over 80%. The fact that such success is due largely to earlier diagnosis is illustrated in an analysis of 103 collections punctured with a fine-needle in a search for pus; only 64 patients had abscesses, 33 of whom were managed subsequently with percutaneously placed drains.[8] Such aggressiveness yields earlier diagnosis and better therapeutic results.

We recently reported a series of 100 patients treated by percutaneous drainage with an 80% cure rate and a 6% mortality rate.[18] This series, added to the evidence of several hundred such procedures already in the literature,[14, 21, 32] now suggests that the majority of abscesses may be managed using small catheters placed percutaneously, with a success rate comparable to that of surgical drainage. Percutaneous drainage has emerged as the procedure of choice.

TECHNIQUES

Imaging

In the majority of patients in whom drainage is performed, cross-sectional imaging is done with the diagnosis of an abscess already suspected. Ultrasonography appears especially useful in subphrenic collections, particularly in patients who have a sympathetic pleural effusion. The diaphragm is well visualized so that a subdiaphragmatic puncture is guaranteed. Often the diaphragm is poorly seen on CT, so that remaining subdiaphragmatic with a needle or catheter may be a problem. Although US is able to localize the majority of abscesses, it often fails with interloop abscesses because of the confusion caused by overlying bowel gas. It may miss some pelvic abscesses for the same reason. Another difficulty with US is the variety of appearances that may be encountered. Usually one sees an echo-poor mass that transmits some sound, but that contains internal echoes. On the other hand, internal gas bubbles may cause a highly echogenic appearance. If air-fluid levels are present, the cavity may be entirely obscured.[6, 16]

Abscesses visualized by CT almost invariably are of low density and, once mature, may have a rim that enhances after IV contrast administration. Gas bubbles are easily seen on current-generation scanners and seldom leave the diagnosis in doubt. Haaga and Weinstein[8] suggested that all suspected abscesses should be punctured with a 22-gauge needle in an attempt to aspirate pus. This certainly confirms the diagnosis and is to be commended; however, intellectual curiosity about a CT finding must be tempered with consideration of the patient's clinical situation and the potential need for drainage.

In some patients, an abscess is an incidental finding, not suspected because leukocytosis and fever are absent. This is perhaps most commonly seen in hepatic abscesses, which may appear simply as a mass on a liver-spleen scan, but subphrenic abscesses also may remain asymptomatic for long periods.

Once an abscess has been visualized, the appropriate position for puncture is marked on the skin while the patient is in the CT scanner, and a clinical decision is then made, after consultation with the appropriate clinicians, whether or not to drain it percutaneously. The first obligation is to decide whether or not the lesion can safely be reached percutaneously. Since a large catheter or drain may be used, this means not violating major abdominal or intrathoracic structures. While we have on occasion drained pseudocysts through the stomach, we would not normally choose to do this, and drainage through any loop of bowel is specifically contraindicated. Nor would we drain through the spleen or liver, although certainly an intrahepatic or intrasplenic catheter may be placed.

The appearance of the abscess itself merely influences one's technique of drainage and seldom produces a contraindication per se. Many abscesses appear to be multilocular on CT, but the majority do not behave as such once a catheter is in position (Fig 9–1).

Dependent drainage is preferred, and it may well be preferable to drain a pelvic abscess surgically through the rectum, rather than uphill with a catheter. This sort of decision is best made in close consultation with the surgical staff.

The route of access is the most important consideration and we feel that it can be best worked out with CT scanning. Usually it is possible to choose a route in the same plane as the lesion, but this is not always the case. In subphrenic abscesses, for example, one certainly would not wish to cross the diaphragm, and thus an uphill puncture is mandated.

With large fluid collections, triangulation is seldom a problem; however,

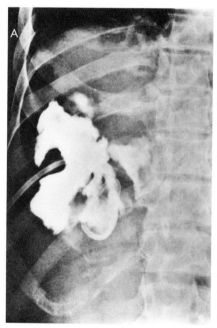
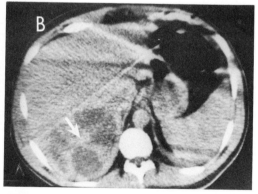

FIG 9–1.
A, the hepatic abscess is drained from a slightly inferior approach to avoid the pleura. The cavity is markedly irregular, but it all appears to be drained from one catheter. **B,** the CT scan before drainage, with the *arrow* pointing to the abscess. The abscess appears to be multilocular, but this was not confirmed by the catheter sinogram. Such an appearance is typical.

localizing small abscesses may be difficult. Computed tomography has certain limitations in this situation, particularly if reconstruction is not available, and US may provide a considerable advantage. Biopsy needles mounted on modi-fied transducers are valuable, but in their absence it is usually simple to localize the lesion with the transducer, "remember" the angle at which one held it, and puncture accordingly.

Puncture

Antibiotic coverage is mandatory for all punctures because of the risk of bac-teremia during the procedure. Antibiotics should be continued, modified by the results of culture and sensitivity.

We perform all punctures under fluoroscopic guidance except for the oc-casional large abscess close to the surface in critically ill patients, in whom the puncture may be performed at the bedside using a trocar technique.

As a rule, however, we puncture the lesion with a 20- or 22-gauge needle, aspirate pus that is sent for Gram stain and culture, and instill a small amount of contrast to confirm the presence of the cavity and to provide an aiming point. We then repuncture with an 18-gauge needle, put in a 0.9-mm wire (0.038-in.), dilate the track, and place a catheter in the traditional Seldinger manner. More recently, and especially if there is a risk of crossing bowel, we have employed the Cope "single-stick" system (Cook Inc., Bloomington, Indi-ana) to avoid two punctures.

It is possible to inject through the catheter while withdrawing over the 0.9-mm wire, and if a loop of bowel has been crossed, the characteristic appearance of intraluminal peristalsing contrast is seen.

Others chose to perform the puncture under CT. It offers an advantage in very difficult punctures, but we find it cumbersome and inconvenient. It shows where the needle has been rather than where it is going, and if one is using the trocar technique one may be at a disadvantage.

On the first day we prefer to place a 10-, 12-, or even 14-French (F) cath-eter, which is coiled in the cavity with a minimum of manipulation (Fig 9–2). Pus is then aspirated for as long as it continues to flow freely. On the first day we try to inject as little contrast as possible so as to avoid bacteremia in an acutely ill patient.

Trocar Technique

Trocar-mounted 8-F pigtail or 14-F sump catheters are available for direct in-sertion (MediTech Inc., Watertown, Massachusetts; Cook Inc.). They are con-venient for US- or CT-monitored drainages but are most useful for large su-perficial collections, which may be drained at the bedside without fluoroscopic guidance. The return of pus signifies a proper catheter position.

MANAGEMENT

Frequently, patients experience defervescence within 24 hours of the initial drainage, although in our experience, patients with hepatic abscess usually re-

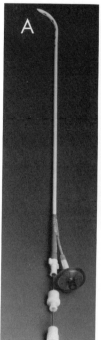
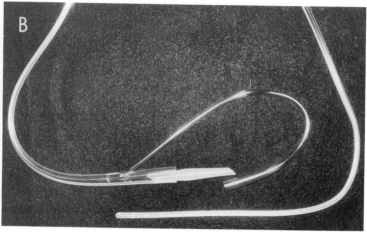

FIG 9–2.

A, a commercially available sump catheter contains a stiffening wire and an optional trocar, so that it may be used for either the trocar or the Seldinger technique. The catheter is manufactured from a biocompatible plastic. The sump lumen is fitted with a microporous bacterial filter. **B,** a Salem sump tube used surgically. The end may be modified with an 18-gauge needle to accept a 0.9-mm guidewire.

quire four or five days for the fever to abate. If the fever persists beyond this time and catheter sinography does not identify separate loculi, a CT scan with contrast injected through the catheter will determine whether or not the entire abscess is being drained. In the face of continued fever or leukocytosis, CT confirmation of adequate drainage mandates the search for a second abscess with a complete CT scan. Traditionally, surgeons have underutilized sinography to ensure that the whole cavity is being drained, and when sinography is combined with cross-sectional imaging, separate noncommunicating abscesses may easily be identified and drained separately. Sinography alone, however, is usually adequate.

Depending on the cavity size, we may elect to exchange for a larger drain at the time of the first sinogram, but in the majority of cases do not exceed 14 F. Single-lumen catheters with multiple sideholes are adequate for small cavities; large cavities may require sump tubes placed on wall suction at 40 to 60 mm Hg. Largely because of the surgeons' familiarity with them, we favor Salem sump tubes, but the specially designed Ring-McLean (Cook Inc.) or vanSonnenberg (MediTech Inc.) sump catheters may be preferable and certainly are softer. Nasogastric tubes with large sideholes circumvent the problem that most sideholes in angiographic catheters are too small.

Occasionally, there will be inadequate drainage through the catheter. Under these circumstances we exchange for a larger sump catheter and use wall suction at 60 mm Hg. We also perform a catheter sinogram to make sure that the catheter is well placed within the cavity. If the problem is due to excessively viscous pus, N-acetyl-cysteine (Mucomyst) may be instilled into the cavity on a regular basis.[2] Occasionally, we have found that a double catheter irrigation system is of use. A small-input catheter is placed (a 5-F pigtail is adequate) and up to 100 ml/hr run into the cavity and aspirated through the sump on suction. Under these circumstances it is critical that the input and output of the cavity are charted so that the patient does not accumulate fluid. It is a technique that can be used only with abscesses with a well-defined outer rim.

The patients are followed up daily by the interventional team, and the catheters are flushed with 5 to 10 ml of saline. Catheter sinograms are performed as necessary. Adequate antibiotics are continued, modified by the growth from the aspirated pus and its sensitivity. The decision to remove the catheter, we think, should be made on clinical grounds.

If the patient is not defervescing, has no undrained loculi, and has an adequate-sized catheter, and if additional abscesses have been excluded, the problem is probably necrotic debris and the approach must be modified (Fig 9–3). Larger catheters are needed and one can dilate the track either with sequential dilations or with an angioplasty balloon catheter to place surgical sumps of 30 or 40 F. We might also place a second catheter and institute an irrigation system with 100 ml/hr flowing through the cavity. N-acetyl-cysteine has been proposed by some to reduce the viscosity of pus and may be successful.[34] In some of these patients surgery will be necessary.

It is important to have a management plan and a series of options worked out well within the time course of the patient's disease. While the objective is to cure patients percutaneously, it is not defensible to persist with inadequate drainage and return a moribund patient to the surgeon. Failures are usually caused by poor catheter technique, but genuine failures must be recognized

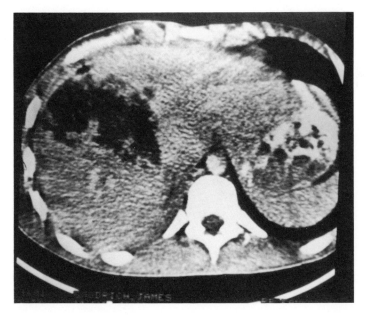

FIG 9–3.
Hepatic abscess. The patient was riding on a motorcycle and struck a deer. The hepatic bleeding was finally controlled by embolization. With such a history, it is not surprising that this cavity contained necrotic debris, and drainage continued for two months before the debris was finally evacuated surgically.

early and these patients operated on while their potential mortality is low.

Early in our experience, we aimed to drain the cavity totally and to see it completely disappear on catheter sinography or CT, but we no longer feel this to be the end point (Fig 9–4). Patients who are not well have incompletely drained abscesses. The same is true of patients with continuing fever and leukocytosis. Once the fever is down and the white blood cell count normal, we begin to look for an opportunity to remove the catheter, which usually comes when drainage ceases. At this point a catheter sinogram is performed and if the cavity is markedly reduced in size, the catheter is removed. Cessation of drainage alone is not an indication for catheter removal. These principles apply to abscesses in almost any location, but details of abscesses in specific areas are discussed separately.

HEPATIC ABSCESSES

The mortality rate for hepatic abscesses has remained high largely because of the difficulty in making the diagnosis. Liver function tests are only mildly disturbed, and if pain does localize to the right upper quadrant, it may be too vague for diagnosis to be certain. With modern imaging methods, however, hepatic abscesses should be diagnosed easily. They may be visible on liver-

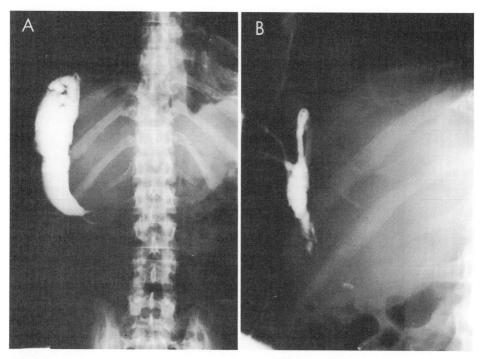

FIG 9–4.
A, a typical subphrenic abscess. **B,** two weeks later, drainage was complete and the catheter could be removed. It should be noted that the approach could have been lower to be sure of avoiding the pleura.

spleen scintigraphy using technetium-labeled sulfur colloid taken up by the reticuloendothelial system, and they are often positive on gallium scanning. We recommend neither method if an abscess is suspected, since their rate of false-negative results is unacceptably high—on the order of 20%. Ultrasonography has greater accuracy, but may miss small, multiple hepatic abscesses, although it should be useful for the associated biliary obstruction, when present.

Computed tomography after contrast administration should have a diagnostic accuracy rate approaching 100%, and with early diagnosis, the mortality rate should fall significantly from 60% to less than 10%.

Amebic Abscesses

Small amebic abscesses respond to metronidazole (Flagyl) and may not need drainage. Larger abscesses probably deserve percutaneous drainage, but it is preferable to empty the cavity and remove the catheter as soon as possible to avoid superinfection. Two to four days of drainage are usually sufficient.[31] The patients are treated with metronidazole during drainage and they tend to experience defervescence quickly. We use an 8-F catheter with multiple sideholes for smaller cavities and a 10- or 12-F catheter for larger cavities. Larger sump tubes are usually not required unless the cavity is very large and an attempt is made to minimize damage to the hepatic parenchyma. Numerous abscesses, when present, are drained with several catheters.

Pyogenic Abscesses

Forty or 50 years ago, the most frequent source of an hepatic abscess was either appendicitis or diverticular disease caused by seeding along the portal vein. Now, hepatic abscesses are more frequently hematogenous although cryptogenic. The majority occur in alcoholic patients, patients with malignant disease or diabetes, or those with biliary disease. Nevertheless, it is surprising how often the etiology remains obscure. Hepatic abscesses are more common in the right lobe and tend to be solitary, although on CT scanning they frequently appear multilocular (see Fig 9–1). Pitt and Zuidema[23] described a higher mortality rate in the elderly (81%), in patients with multiple abscesses (88%), and in those treated with either antibiotics alone or surgery alone (97%). It is of interest that the frequency of hepatic abscesses has not declined despite the widespread use of antibiotics.[11]

Once drainage is initiated, it is important to be sure that the catheter sinogram corresponds to the appearance on the other imaging modalities and that no loculus is being overlooked. We have found that patients tend to defervesce on the fourth or fifth day if drainage is adequate. In our first seven patients, the average hospital stay was three weeks.[17] Now it is closer to two weeks, which compares favorably with the six weeks necessary for recuperation after surgical treatment.[24]

Multiple hepatic abscesses are most often associated with biliary obstruction, and transhepatic cholangiography may be required to identify or exclude such obstruction. If possible, each loculus should be drained, and the biliary system may need to be decompressed. There is also an entity of multiple microabscesses associated with biliary obstruction; this is usually fatal and can be managed only by antibiotics and biliary decompression, as the abscesses are too small for individual drainage. It is effectively a variant of ascending cholangitis.

We have also seen focal microabscesses occupying one hepatic segment for which drainage was unsuccessful (Fig 9–5). The one patient we encountered died on the second day, and there is another reported death of such a patient.[33] Perhaps in the future we should recommend surgery in these patients, but we are not sanguine with respect to the outcome.

Our results with 20 hepatic abscesses are similar to our overall results of abscess drainage. Except for reluctance to rely on percutaneous drainage for focal microabscesses, the treatment and management are the same as for abscesses in general.[10] R. B. Dietrick (personal communication, 1981), in Korea, reported the largest experience. Seventy-four patients were treated with antibiotics and surgical drainage, with a mortality rate of 12%; 99 patients were treated percutaneously by repeated aspirations (average, 5) rather than by catheter drainage, with three deaths (mortality rate, 3%). Catheter drainage would have been an improvement. It appeared in that series to make little difference whether the lesions were pyogenic or amebic.

SUBPHRENIC AND INTRA-ABDOMINAL ABSCESSES

Most subphrenic and intra-abdominal abscesses occur postoperatively, frequently after surgery for a perforated bowel. Subphrenic abscesses are usually easier to drain, but may require 15- or 20-F catheters if the cavities are large (over 1 L). Drainage time is usually about two weeks, but if there is an associ-

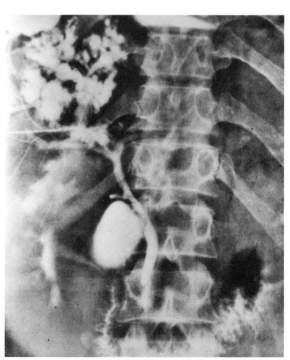

FIG 9–5.
The most virulent form of hepatic abscess. The appearances are suggestive of microabscesses, frequently associated with biliary obstruction, but they are localized to one segment. For this reason, cholangiography was performed to exclude biliary obstruction. Although drainage of both the abscess and the biliary system was undertaken, the patient died within 48 hours.

ated fistula, it must be controlled, which will add to the time. Subphrenic abscesses are easily visualized on both US and CT, but US has an advantage in that the diaphragm can easily be defined and the route of access kept below it. Occasionally, a large sympathetic pleural effusion makes it difficult to distinguish clinically between an empyema and a subphrenic abscess. The question may be resolved by inserting a needle into the two spaces, but great care must be taken not to contaminate the uninfected space.

Interloop abscesses are more difficult to drain and may be very difficult to visualize. Ultrasonography is poor, but good CT scanning is successful so long as all the bowel loops are opacified. It requires meticulous technique. It is especially important not to perforate the bowel, and injecting contrast while withdrawing the needle or catheter over a guidewire may be a useful maneuver. If there is a drain track, we have occasionally been successful with steerable MediTech catheters. If there is an enteric leak, all the loculi of the abscess must be drained, sometimes separately, and a controlled fistula developed. Occasionally, it is not possible to reach an interloop abscess safely, and operation must be advised.

ENTERIC FISTULAS

Enteric fistulas are perhaps the most challenging collections to drain, but it is possible to control a lateral duodenal or even an end duodenal fistula.[19, 28] Control of the output of the pancreas and the biliary system in addition to the succus entericus requires exact positioning of several catheters. If access is difficult, it may be possible to negotiate drain tracks using steerable MediTech systems. Once a catheter is in position, catheter sinography is critical and may delineate multiple fistulous tracks into secondary cavities, all of which must be drained.

The various outputs may amount to several liters per day. Managing the patient's metabolic demands is vitally important and requires close cooperation with the surgical staff. It may be useful to place a T-tube in the bowel through the tract so as to divert the enteric stream, at least partially.[20] The aim is to develop a controlled fistula and to dry up the site of previous leaks.[15] It may be advantageous to enter and drain the biliary system separately. Drainage of this sort requires several months and obviously necessitates concomitant parenteral nutrition, but it is preferable, at least in some instances, to surgery, which even today carries a high mortality of the order of 25%.[30] If complete control cannot be achieved, early surgery is necessary.

More distal enteric fistulas require the same amount of care and precision in catheter placement, but are less demanding because the volume loss is less and the fistulous systems are fewer. Again, the objective is to develop a controlled fistula in an otherwise dry bed and then to allow the fistula to close.

PELVIC ABSCESSES

Because the basic principle of dependent drainage should be considered, many pelvic abscesses are best drained in the traditional surgical manner, through the rectum or vagina. If the abscesses are a little higher, they may also be drained percutaneously. The problem is one of a safe approach, which is best planned by CT scanning. Ultrasonography may be unreliable, and a fluid-filled loop of bowel, unseen during sonography, may intervene between the skin and the catheter. If a safe route of access is unavailable, the patient should be managed surgically, but when percutaneous drainage has been instituted, we have been as successful with abscesses located in the pelvis as with those elsewhere. Enteric leaks need separate control. If the urinary tract is perforated, upper urinary tract diversion by nephrostomy is also required. The site of the urinary fistula should be delineated by antegrade studies and, if it is in the ureter, the transected ureter should be crossed and stented. Fistulas involving only the bladder can probably be managed either by Foley catheter drainage or suprapubic drainage; if this proves inadequate, bilateral nephrostomies will be required.

PANCREATIC COLLECTIONS

It appears that our terminology is outmoded and we are just beginning to classify and label the new information we have obtained from US and CT. There seems to be too much new information to fit too few old labels. Pseudocysts were well defined in the surgical literature as palpable lesions found weeks or months after an episode of pancreatitis. They have been drained largely because of their size and associated pressure symptoms, coupled with fears of their rupture. Pancreatic abscesses have been found when patients with acute hemorrhagic pancreatitis were operated on or died. They were assumed to be related to the very high mortality of acute pancreatitis and were perhaps its most virulent complication. Only about 5% of patients with pancreatitis develop abscesses, however. Pseudocysts and abscesses are therefore surgical terms based on clinical findings.

Now that US and CT are performed frequently on patients with pancreatitis, we have discovered that collections are common and often come and go.[29] Pseudocysts in the literature on CT are defined as well-circumscribed collections with nonenhancing rims (Fig 9–6). They may regress spontaneously and may be silent clinically. Abscesses are indistinguishable from other ragged-looking collections and may involve the lesser sac or retroperitoneum. Gerzof and associates[7] suggested that pseudocysts should be classified as infected and noninfected on the basis of fine-needle puncture and Gram's stain, and that collections be so divided also. Infected collections may be called abscesses and infected pseudocysts may be called infected pseudocysts (not abscesses). They recommend drainage only for the infected lesions.[7] This approach is at least logical.

Pancreatic Abscesses

We have drained seven pancreatic lesions. They yielded *Escherichia coli, Klebsiella pneumoniae, Proteus mirabilis*, and *Pseudomonas*, sometimes in mixed culture (Fig 9–7). The amylase level in the fluid was usually high (20,000 to 40,000 IU/

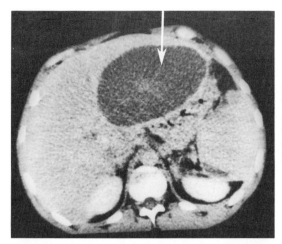

FIG 9–6.
Typical CT appearance of a pseudocyst
(arrow). This patient is unusual in that
the pseudocyst is anterior to the
stomach. Drainage was successfully
terminated within five days.

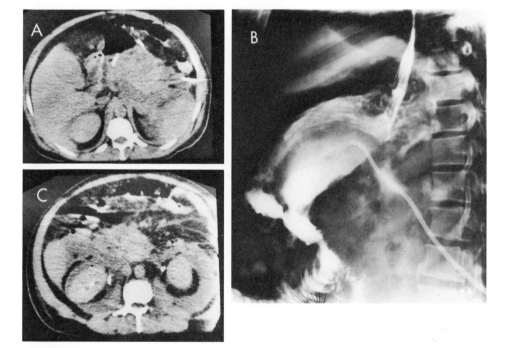

FIG 9–7.
A, seven days after an attack of acute hemorrhagic pancreatitis, the patient was seen with a lesser
sac abscess. The drainage catheter is visible. **B,** location of the lesser sac is well demonstrated, with
the stomach being displaced forward. One can also see anterior displacement of the lesser sac by
the bulging retroperitoneum. **C,** a CT scan lower in the same patient shows extensive collections in
the anterior and posterior pararenal spaces that were not drained separately. Such extensive collections are seen not infrequently now that CT is being performed regularly in patients with severe
pancreatitis.

ml). In all patients we drained the lesser sac, as this was the most approachable collection, and in three patients set up a double-irrigation system. Such a system may share some of the advantages of peritoneal lavage advocated by some authors for acute pancreatitis.[27, 35] All patients showed initial improvement, but drainage appeared to be incomplete due to necrotic debris in three patients, and they were operated on. One of these patients had been deteriorating over the last ten days of a 40-day drainage period and died of respiratory failure following surgery. In retrospect, surgery should not have been delayed so long. One other patient died of renal and respiratory failure, although it appeared that drainage had caused defervescence.[13]

From our experience, we continue to recommend percutaneous drainage of pancreatic abscesses; however, since it was curative in only half of the patients, it should be regarded as palliative. Two of our patients required both respiratory and circulatory support before drainage. Once the patient's condition begins to improve, any further deterioration should be a signal for immediate surgical intervention.

We have also seen patients with large retroperitoneal collections that on needling appeared to represent only edema and from which no fluid could be obtained. We believe an aggressive approach is to be encouraged, since pancreatic abscesses carry a mortality rate on the order of 70% or 80%[25]; but our experience and that of others at this stage is only preliminary.

Pseudocysts

We offer percutaneous drainage of enlarging, symptomatic pseudocysts as an alternative for patients in whom surgery was planned. We keep drainage to an average of eight days in an attempt to avoid superinfection. Percutaneous needle evacuation of pseudocysts, which has been practiced for some years, carries a significant recurrence rate and we hope catheter drainage is an improvement.

Hancke and Pedersen[9] reported on 14 cases drained with an 18-gauge needle, with primary success in 14 but a recurrence rate of 50% in one year. We had no recurrences at one year, but since then have seen two recurrences out of nine patients, both at 15 months. It is possible that in chronic disease such as pancreatitis these may have been new pseudocysts in a similar location.

The suggestion by Gerzof and associates[7] that only infected pseudocysts be drained percutaneously seems to be reasonable and conservative. Surgeons do operate on uninfected pseudocysts, however, and percutaneous management may appear preferable to surgery. It must be remembered that even the largest pseudocyst will occasionally resolve spontaneously.

Results

We recently reported the results of abscess drainage in 100 patients, of whom eight had multiple abscesses and the most in any one patient was six.[18] The distribution of the abscesses is as follows:

Subphrenic and intra-abdominal	37
Hepatic	20 (4 amebic)
Pancreatic and pancreatic pseudocysts	16
Pelvic	8
Retroperitoneal	6
Renal and perineal	5
Other (including mediastinal)	8

As can be seen, the majority were intra-abdominal; three were in the mediastinum. The overall cure rate for the series was 85%, and the average drainage time in the last 50 patients was reduced to two weeks.

The failure rate of 15% is worth considering specifically (Table 9–1). Four of these patients had early surgery before the results of drainage could be assessed, and a fifth patient was operated on for an infected hepatic cyst. A sixth patient had a hepatoma that appeared to be a recurrent abscess, and two patients, one with an enteric fistula and the other with a subphrenic abscess, were inadequately drained early in our experience through poor radiologic technique. One final patient had a pseudocyst that did not collapse with drainage; indeed it felt rather like a tennis ball when it was punctured, and he underwent a distal pancreatectomy. Six patients, therefore, had inadequate treatment and represent the failure of the technique of percutaneous drainage. Three patients died.

It is reasonable to suppose, therefore, that a cure rate of at least 90% is

TABLE 9–1.

Causes of Failure of Drainage

LOCATION	ETIOLOGY	DRAINAGE PERIOD (WK)	REASON FOR FAILURE
Hepatic	Unknown	2 days	Died
Pancreatic	Hemorrhagic pancreatitis	6	Necrotic debris, recurrent infection (died)
Pancreatic	Hemorrhagic pancreatitis	2	Necrotic debris
Pancreatic	Hemorrhagic pancreatitis	7	Necrotic debris
Pseudocyst	Chronic pancreatitis	5 days	Would not collapse
Hepatic	Cholangiocarcinoma	4	Carcinoma (died)
Hepatic	Post-traumatic	12	Necrotic debris
Hepatic	Cyst	1	Became infected, early surgery
Hepatic	Hepatoma presenting as recurrent abscess	2	Hepatoma
Subphrenic	Postoperative	2	Inadequate drainage
Intraperitoneal	Anastomotic leak (postoperative)	2	Inadequate drainage
Intraperitoneal	Anastomotic leak (postoperative)	1	Inadequate drainage
Pancreatic	Postoperative	6 days	Early surgery
Pancreatic	Postoperative	1 day	Early surgery
Pancreatic	Hemorrhagic pancreatitis	1 day	Early surgery

achievable. These numbers deserve close scrutiny because failures of drainage represent potential deaths, since the mortality for untreated abscesses approaches 100%. For the percutaneous technique to be justifiable, such patients must be recognized early and be operated on while the chance for a cure remains high. From the examination of our failures, enteric leaks and patients with necrotic debris, particularly in the pancreas, are the most likely to fail a trial of percutaneous drainage. A more aggressive approach involving dilatation to place 30- to 40-F catheters and the use of a double-irrigation system might be more rewarding in patients with necrotic debris, but there is no direct evidence that this will be so.

Our series mortality rate, when defined as a 30-day mortality, was 6%. One of these patients with a multiloculated hepatic abscess was admitted in gram-negative septicemia and died on the second day. A second patient had a pancreatic abscess and was drained while intubated and receiving dopamine support. She was palliated for 30 days but was not operated on as soon as her condition deteriorated, and she died postoperatively. (She died on the 40th day but is included in our statistics.) A third death was a patient with extensive cholangiocarcinoma and multiple hepatic abscesses who died on the 30th day after drainage, as much from carcinoma as from sepsis. There were three other deaths within 30 days that did not appear to be associated in that the patients were not infected, but had malignancies. Indeed, there was no catheter in place in two of these patients. In all, 12 patients died in the group of 100 patients from two days to nine months after initiating percutaneous drainage. Half of them had malignant disease.

Collating our experience with three large series from the literature (Gerzof,[5] 67 patients; vanSonnenberg and colleagues,[33] 51 patients; and Haaga and Weinstein,[8] 33 patients), 251 abscesses were drained percutaneously for a mortality rate of less than 5% and a cure rate of greater than 80%. A typical surgical series is 100 subphrenic abscesses with a mortality rate of 30%.[1] This series is by no means comparable, however, since almost certainly the diagnosis is being made much earlier today because of the prevalence and success of CT scanning.

CONCLUSION

From our experience and that of others, large-bore catheters are not necessary to drain the majority of abscesses; 14 F suffices for most lesions. Should larger catheters be necessary because of the presence of necrotic debris, they can be introduced percutaneously by prior dilatation of the track with an angioplasty catheter. We favor sump tubes, but probably any catheter with large sideholes is adequate. The most common cause of inadequate drainage seems to be poor radiologic technique. The second most common cause of failure is the presence of a second abscess that is unsuspected and therefore undrained. True failures of drainage must be recognized early and operated on.

It is the close involvement of the radiologist, most specifically diagnostically but also therapeutically, that has led to the lowering of mortality rates of abscess drainage, a disease that is certainly not decreasing in frequency. Palliative drainage may be all that is possible in some instances, such as pancreatic abscesses or enteric fistulas, and the technique should be employed judiciously. From the results in the literature so far (over 300 patients), percutaneous drainage would appear to be the procedure of first choice and we recognize only one major contraindication: inability to reach the lesion safely.

REFERENCES

1. Bonfils-Roberts EA, Barone JE, Nealson RF: Treatment of subphrenic abscesses. *Surg Clin North Am* 1975; 55:1361.
2. Dawson SL, Mueller PR, Ferrucci JT Jr: Mucomyst for abscesses: A clinical comment. *Radiology* 1984; 151:342.
3. Decosse JJ, et al: Subphrenic abscess. *Surg Gynecol Obstet* 1974; 138:841–849.
4. Gerzof SG, et al: Percutaneous catheter drainage of abdominal abscesses guided by ultrasound and computed tomography. *AJR* 1979; 133:1–8.
5. Gerzof SG, et al: Percutaneous catheter drainage of abdominal abscesses: A 5-year experience. *N Engl J Med* 1981; 305:653–657.
6. Gerzof SG: Ultrasound in the search for abdominal abscesses. *Clin Diagn Ultrasound* 1981; 7:101–106.
7. Gerzof SG, et al: The role of percutaneous aspiration on drainage in the diagnosis and therapy of acute pancreatitis. Presented at the Radiological Society of North America. Chicago, November 1981.
8. Haaga JR, Weinstein AJ: CT-guided percutaneous aspiration and drainage of abscesses. *AJR* 1980; 135:1187–1194.
9. Hancke S, Pedersen JR: Percutaneous puncture of pancreatic cysts guided by ultrasound. *Surg Gynecol Obstet* 1976; 142:551–552.
10. Johnson RD, et al: Percutaneous drainage of pyogenic liver abscesses. *AJR* 1985; 144:463–467.
11. Joseph WL, Kahn AM, Longmire WP: Pyogenic liver abscess. *Am Surg* 1978; 115:63–68.
12. Karlson KB, et al: Percutaneous abscess drainage. *Surg Gynecol Obstet* 1982; 154:44–48.
13. Karlson KB, et al: Percutaneous drainage of pancreatic pseudocysts and abscesses. *Radiology* 1982; 142:619–624.
14. Keller FS, et al: Percutaneous interventional catheter therapy for lesions of the chest and lungs. *Chest* 1982; 81:407–412.
15. Kerlan RK, et al: Abdominal abscess with low-output fistula: Successful percutaneous drainage. *Radiology* 1985; 155:73–75.
16. Kressel HY, Filly RA: Ultrasonographic appearance of gas-containing abscesses in the abdomen. *AJR* 1978; 130:71–73.
17. Martin EC, et al: Percutaneous drainage in the management of hepatic abscesses. *Surg Clin North Am* 1981; 61:157–167.
18. Martin EC, Fankuchen EI, Neff RA: Percutaneous drainage of abscess: A report of 100 patients. *Clin Radiol* 1983; 35:9–11.
19. McFadzean AJS, Chang KPS, Wong CC: Solitary pyogenic abscess of the liver treated by closed aspiration and antibiotics: A report of 14 consecutive cases with recovery. *Br J Surg* 1953; 41:141–152.
20. McLean GK, et al: Enterocutaneous fistulae: Interventional radiologic management. *AJR* 1982; 138:615–619.
21. Mueller PR, vanSonnenberg E, Ferrucci JT Jr: Percutaneous drainage of 250 ab-

dominal abscesses and fluid collections: II. Current procedural concepts. *Radiology* 1984; 151:343–347.

22. Ochsner A, DeBakey M, Murray S: Pyogenic abscesses of the liver: Part 2. *Am J Surg* 1948; 40:292–319.
23. Pitt HA, Zuidema CD: Factors influencing mortality in the treatment of pyogenic hepatic abscess. *Surg Gynecol Obstet* 1975; 140:228–234.
24. Ranson JHC, et al: New diagnostic and therapeutic techniques in the management of pyogenic liver abscesses. *Ann Surg* 1975; 181:508–518.
25. Ranson JHC, et al: Prognostic signal and the role of operative management in acute pancreatitis. *Surg Gynecol Obstet* 1976; 143:209.
26. Ranson JHC: Acute pancreatitis. *Surg Clin North Am* 1981; 61:55–70.
27. Ranson JHC, Spencer FC: The role of peritoneal lavage in severe acute pancreatitis. *Ann Surg* 1978; 187:656–662.
28. Rogers L: Lettsomian lectures on amoebic liver abscess. *Lancet* 1922; 2:1463–1468, 1569–1576, 1677–1682.
29. Siegelman SS, et al: CT of fluid collection as associated with pancreatitis. *AJR* 1980; 134:1121–1132.
30. Soeter PB, Ebeid AM, Fischer JE: Review of 404 patients with gastrointestinal fistulas. *Ann Surg* 1979; 190:189–202.
31. vanSonnenberg E, et al: Intrahepatic amebic abscesses: Indications for and results of percutaneous catheter drainage. *Radiology* 1985; 156:631–635.
32. vanSonnenberg E, Mueller PR, Ferrucci JT Jr: Percutaneous drainage of 250 abdominal abscesses and fluid collections: I. Results, failures and complications. *Radiology* 1984; 151:337–341.
33. vanSonnenberg E, et al: Percutaneous drainage of abscesses and fluid collections: Techniques, results and applications. *Radiology* 1982; 142:1–10.
34. van Waes PFGM, et al: Management of loculated abscesses that are difficult to drain: A new approach. *Radiology* 1983; 147:37–63.
35. Wall AJP: Peritoneal dialysis in the treatment of severe acute pancreatitis. *Med J Aust* 1965; 2:281–289.
36. Yates JL: An experimental study of the local effects of peritoneal drainage. *Surg Gynecol Obstet* 1905; 1:473–481.

10

Percutaneous Biopsy and Drainage of Pelvic Masses

Janis G. Letourneau, M.D.

Masses within the pelvis can arise from a number of anatomic structures, including the gastrointestinal tract, bladder, lymph nodes, muscle, bone, the uterus and ovaries in the female, and the prostate and seminal vesicles in the male. The character of many of these masses can be determined on the basis of percutaneous biopsy. Diagnostic and therapeutic drainage of abnormal fluid collections in the pelvis can also often be performed percutaneously.

LOCALIZATION

The most precise means of localization for biopsy or drainage of pelvic masses is usually computed tomography (CT). This is primarily due to the fact that CT imaging is not as adversely affected by the presence of bowel in the pelvis as is ultrasound (US). It also easily permits examination of the patient in a variety of positions, optimizing the planning and performance of percutaneous procedures. Thus, many patients may be scanned in a prone position, permitting an extraperitoneal approach to biopsy and drainage.[1] Localization with US for pelvic procedures is often limited by the need for distention of the urinary bladder to provide an adequate anterior acoustic window; a transgluteal approach has alternatively been utilized for US of the posterior pelvis.[7] Ultrasound can, therefore, be useful in guidance of selected cases and is especially valuable in renal transplant patients and in those patients requiring bedside diagnostic or therapeutic aspirations of pelvic fluid collections.

Fluoroscopic guidance for percutaneous pelvic procedures is limited primarily to biopsy of lymph nodes following lymphangiography. Fluoroscopy, of course, is often of value in directing catheter and guidewire manipulations in a drainage procedure, once localization has been accomplished with CT or US.

BIOPSY

Once the target lesion has been localized, the path of the biopsy needle must be precisely determined. If CT guidance has been used, the angle and depth of needle placement can be obtained directly from the scanner electronics (Fig 10–1,A). If an anterior approach is planned and if there is a likelihood of traversing bowel loops, a fine needle should be used. A posterior puncture site, however, often provides excellent access to a pelvic mass and permits somewhat greater flexibility in needle selection (Fig 10–1,B). Frequently, a large cutting-type needle such as a Tru-Cut can be used in this setting (Fig 10–2). Although lymph nodes have been traditionally biopsied with fluoroscopic guidance following lymphangiographic opacification,[3–5, 9] lymph node biopsy can be accomplished without opacification following CT or US localization (Fig 10–3).

DRAINAGE OF PELVIC FLUID COLLECTIONS

Pelvic fluid collections, similar to fluid collections in other locations, can be free or loculated. They can have various compositions, being serous, purulent, hemorrhagic, or lymphatic in nature. Therapeutic aspiration of these collections may be of value in the management of patients and can be performed with CT or US guidance (Fig 10–4,A and B). Guidance with CT is often preferred for drainage of most pelvic collections, although US guidance can also be used, particularly for large or superficial collections. Computed tomographic guidance provides precise information on the location of bowel loops, a factor more important in catheter drainage procedures than in biopsy procedures, as a catheter should not be placed through a bowel loop. Computed tomographic guidance permits planning of an extraperitoneal catheter tract from the more desirable anterior approach[12] and also from a posterior approach.

RESULTS AND COMPLICATIONS

Specific statistics on results of percutaneous biopsy in the pelvis are difficult to separate from those of biopsy in the abdomen. Some reported series are, however, limited to diagnostic problems in the pelvis. The value of CT-guided biopsy in the setting of previous resection for rectal carcinoma has been clearly established.[1, 6, 10, 11, 14] In one series, percutaneous biopsy was diagnostic of recurrence or infection in 19 of 28 patients who underwent such a procedure. The accuracy rate for recurrence was higher than these numbers indicate, with 15 of 19 solid lesions positive for recurrence and with four of 19 solid lesions demonstrating true-negative biopsy pathology.[1] In a study performed on pa-

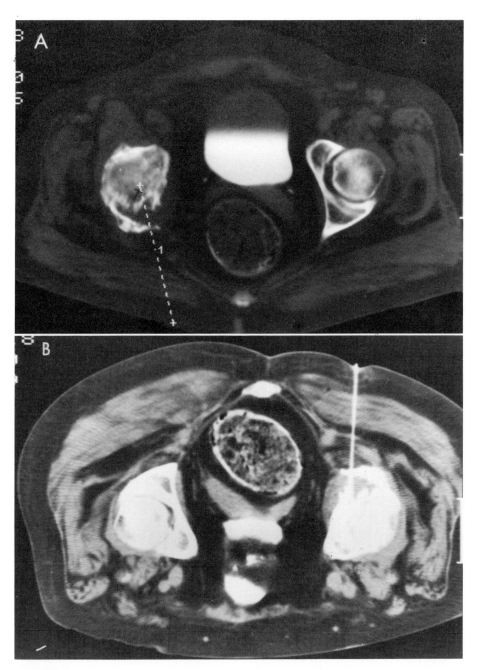

FIG 10–1.
A, determination of the needle course and depth using the CT scanner calculations in the setting of a bony metastasis in a patient with metastatic carcinoma of unknown primary. **B,** the patient was placed in a prone position for CT-guided needle biopsy of the lytic lesion of the acetabulum.

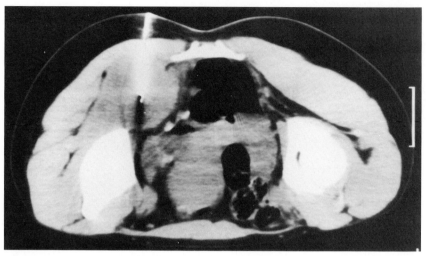

FIG 10–2.
This large soft-tissue mass, a rhabdomyosarcoma located in the posterior pelvis, was biopsied with a 14-gauge Tru-Cut needle from a posterior approach.

tients with known gynecological malignancies, 66% of the percutaneous biopsies performed were successful in providing a diagnosis. All but one of the biopsies performed involved masses that were pelvic in location.[8] A series of fluoroscopically guided percutaneous biopsies of lymph nodes in patients with cervical carcinoma revealed an overall accuracy of 68% and a predictive value of 100% for a positive test.[3] These series all emphasize the limited value of a negative biopsy result in the setting of known malignancy.

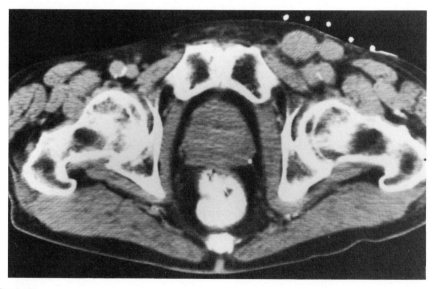

FIG 10–3.
Final localization of enlarged inguinal nodes in a patient with lymphoma was accomplished using a series of radiopaque catheters taped into a linear arrangement.

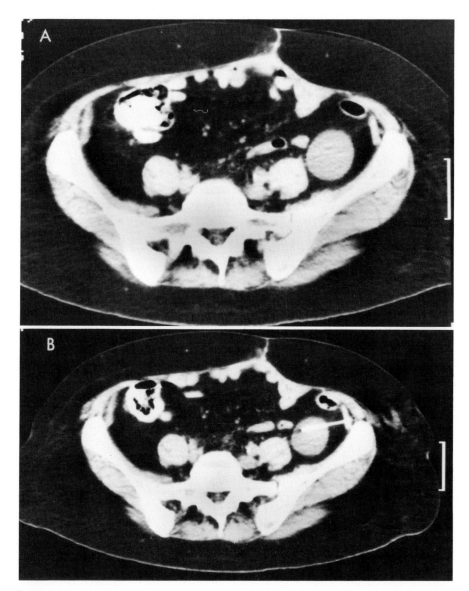

FIG 10–4.
A, a fluid collection was identified in the left lower quadrant of this patient with endometrial carcinoma following hysterectomy and surgical staging. **B,** therapeutic drainage of this lymphocele was performed with CT-guidance by simple aspiration with a 20-gauge needle.

The impact of percutaneous drainage of pelvic fluid collections on patient care is also great. Again, the results of these procedures are often reported in larger series of abdominal drainages. Some special situations, however, deserve mention. In a series of patients with iliopsoas abscess, seven of eight percutaneous drainages were successful.[12] Percutaneous drainage of pelvic lymphoceles has also been shown to be effective, with nine of 11 patients in one report cured by simple aspiration or catheter drainage.[13] Despite the complex clinical circumstances that frequently are present in relation to transplant patients, the value of percutaneous drainage of perinephric fluid collections is clearly established.[2] The drainage may not be therapeutically definitive, however, as surgical correction of the primary problem may still be required.

Complications are infrequently seen in conjunction with biopsy or drainage of pelvic masses. Most biopsy series describe no significant complications.[3, 4] The Massachusetts General Hospital report of percutaneous biopsy in 28 patients who had undergone surgery for rectal carcinoma noted one significant complication, gross hematuria requiring transfusion.[1] Seeding of a pelvic fluid collection seems to be the most significant complication of percutaneous drainage, with secondary infection of hematoma[2] and colonization of lymphoceles being described occasionally.[13]

CONCLUSION

The pelvis is a complex anatomic space that can be precisely examined with newer imaging modalities. Computed tomography and US provide excellent means of target lesion localization for biopsy and drainage of pelvic masses. Fluoroscopic guidance is valuable in the setting of lymph node biopsy and for catheter and guidewire manipulations.

REFERENCES

1. Butch RJ, Wittenberg J, Mueller PR, et al: Presacral masses after abdominoperineal resection for colorectal carcinoma: The need for needle biopsy. *AJR* 1985; 144:308–312.
2. Curry NS, Cochran S, Barbaric Z, et al: Interventional radiologic procedures in the renal transplant. *Radiology* 1984; 152:647–653.
3. Edeiken-Monroe BS, Zornoza J: Carcinoma of the cervix: Percutaneous lymph node aspiration biopsy. *AJR* 1982; 138:655–657.
4. Efremidis SC, Dan SJ, Nieburgs H, et al: Carcinoma of the prostate: Lymph node aspiration for staging. *AJR* 1984; 136:489–492.
5. Gothlin JH, Holem L: Percutaneous fine-needle biopsy of radiographically normal lymph nodes in the staging of prostatic carcinoma. *Radiology* 1985; 141:351–354.
6. Grabbe E, and Winkler R: Local recurrence after sphincter-saving resection for rectal and rectosigmoid carcinoma: Value of various diagnostic methods. *Radiology* 1985; 155:305–310.
7. Heckemann R, Wernecke K, Hagel J, et al: Transgluteal sonography: A new approach to the posterior pelvic compartment. *Radiology* 1983; 147:587–589.
8. Jaques PF, Staab E, Richey W, et al: CT-assisted pelvic and abdominal aspiration biopsies in gynecological malignancy. *Radiology* 1978; 128:651–655.
9. Kidd R, Correa R Jr: Fine-needle aspiration biopsy of lymphangiographically normal lymph nodes: A negative view. *AJR* 1984; 141:1005–1006.
10. Lee JKT, Stanley RJ, Sagel SS, et al: CT appearance of the pelvis after abdominoperineal resection for rectal carcinoma. *Radiology* 1981; 141:737–741.
11. McCarthy SM, Barnes D, DeVeney K, et al: Detection of recurrent rectosigmoid carcinoma: Prospective evaluation of CT and clinical factors. *AJR* 1985; 144:577–579.

12. Mueller PR, Ferrucci JT Jr, Wittenberg J, et al: Iliopsoas abscess: Treatment by CT-guided percutaneous catheter drainage. *AJR* 1984; 142:359–362.
13. White M, Mueller PR, Ferrucci JT Jr, et al: Percutaneous drainage of postoperative abdominal and pelvic lymphoceles. *AJR* 1985; 145:1065–1069.
14. Zelas P, Haaga JR, Lavery IC, et al: The diagnosis by percutaneous biopsy with computed tomography of a recurrence of carcinoma of the rectum in the pelvis. *Surg Gynecol Obstet* 1980; 151:525–527.

11

Aspirations Performed for Miscellaneous Conditions

Morteza K. Elyaderani, M.D.

BIOPSY OF BREAST LESIONS

Localization of Nonpalpable Breast Masses

Nonpalpable breast lesions are being detected more frequently because of advances in mammographic techniques. Biopsy of indeterminate lesions can be directed by noninvasive or invasive localization techniques. Estimation of the lesion site and its depth can be made directly from the mammogram. This is only adequate for superficial or periareolar lesions. More precise localization can be made by the insertion of radiopaque markers in proximity to the lesions.

Surface Method Localization

This method is noninvasive and provides a "map" of the relative position of the suspicious area within the breast. The distance from the lesion to the nipple is measured in the vertical and horizontal axes, using the mediolateral and craniocaudal mammograms for reference. The method lacks precision, as it is only accurate when the breast is in the same position as when the mammogram was performed. The lesion would be expected to shift its relative position within the breast when the patient is in a supine position for surgery.

The Spot Method

The spot technique for breast lesion localization utilizes radiographic contrast and vital stains. The distance of the lesion from the nipple along horizontal and vertical planes is measured from the mediolateral and craniocaudal views of the mammogram, respectively. The depth of the lesion is determined from either view and these measurements are transferred to the patient's breast, with the patient sitting as she would be for mammography. This can even be done with breast compression. The x- and y-axes are drawn, using the nipple as the center point. The vertical distance from the nipple is marked on the y-axis. From this point, a line is drawn parallel to the x-axis (Fig 11–1,A). The horizontal distance from the nipple is marked on the x-axis and from this point a line is drawn parallel to the y-axis for needle insertion (Fig 11–1,B). The point where these two lines cross is the needle insertion site (Fig 11–1,C). This method is not accurate when the lesion is deep or if the breast is large and pendulous, because of the curvature of the breast surface. In these cases the distance from the nipple to the marked point on the skin will be too short because of using straight lines to measure from the nipple along the horizontal and vertical axes. To resolve this problem, the arc method can be used. In this technique, the distance from the nipple along the horizontal and vertical axes is measured from mediolateral and craniocaudal mammograms along the breast curvature (Fig 11–2).

The point selected on the skin for needle puncture should define a tract to the lesion perpendicular to the skin surface or parallel to the chest wall. The needle is then inserted along this tract. At least two factors should be considered prior to transferring the mammographic measurements to the patient's breast: magnification and compression. Without correction for magnification the direct measurements taken from the mammogram will overestimate the distance of the lesion from the nipple in both horizontal and vertical axes. Correction must also take into account breast positioning and compression, factors that will depend on the specific mammographic unit being used.

A 22- to 25-gauge needle of sufficient length is adequate for localization. Use of a fine-needle with deep lesions may not be desirable, because of difficulty with placement secondary to needle flexibility. After determining the puncture site on the patient's skin, the needle is advanced to the predetermined depth. The position of its tip is determined by two mammographic views. If the needle is not in an acceptable location, its position is readjusted and another set of mammograms is obtained. When the needle tip is positioned in the desired location, 0.5 to 1.0 ml of methylene blue or Evan's blue and an approximately equal amount of radiopaque water-soluble contrast are injected and postinjection mammograms are obtained.[5, 15, 17, 30, 31] The contrast material and dye act as landmarks to guide the surgeon during biopsy. One may inject additional methylene or Evan's blue along the tract as the needle is removed to further aid the surgeon.[5]

An advantage of the spot technique is that the needle is not the surgical marker, and therefore accidental needle displacement will not invalidate the lesion localization. The major disadvantage of this technique is that if the first spot is not properly injected, a second spot cannot be injected without causing confusion for the radiologist and surgeon. Another disadvantage is that the dye gradually diffuses within the breast parenchyma, so biopsy should be performed as soon as possible (within 0.5 to four hours). If the dye enters ducts within the breast parenchyma, even more rapid dispersion is seen. This technique has been shown to be accurate and safe.[5, 15, 30]

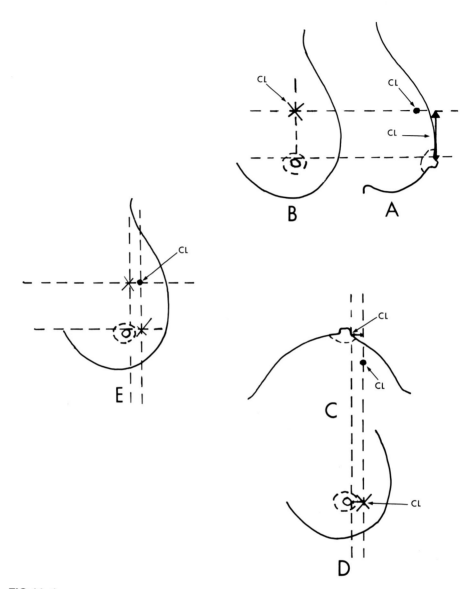

FIG 11–1.
Linear technique. **A,** a schematic mediolateral mammogram shows a lesion *(dark spot–arrow)* to be localized. The vertical distance from the nipple to the lesion is measured *(arrow).* **B,** this measurement is transferred to the breast and is marked on the skin *(arrow).* **C,** a schematic craniocaudal mammogram of breast shows the lesion *(dark spot)* and its horizontal distance from the nipple is measured *(arrow).* **D,** the horizontal measurement is transferred over the breast and is marked on the patient's skin. **E,** vertical and horizontal lines from the two marks on the patient's skin are drawn parallel to the vertical and horizontal lines of measurements from the nipple. These two lines are crossing each other on the skin over the lesion. *CL* = crossing lines.

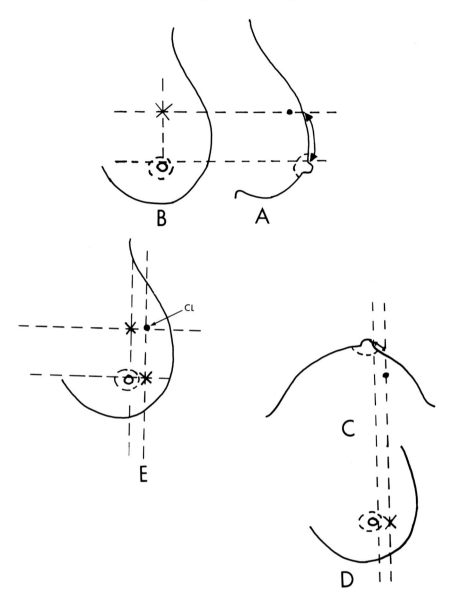

FIG 11–2.
A–E, arch technique. The technique is similar to the linear technique, but the distance of lesion from the nipple along the horizontal and vertical lines is measured along the breast curvature.

Localization by Needle

To localize by needle, dye is not injected following needle insertion. Instead the needle is secured in place with a strip of tape, following mammographic documentation of proximity of the needle tip to the lesion.[4, 23] If the tip is more than 2 cm from the lesion, a second needle is inserted using the first needle as a guide. Mammograms are repeated. Repeat mammography after introduction of the needle may cause needle displacement. To minimize displacement the needle must be inserted to its hub or be taped securely.

Self-Retaining Wire Localization

A specially designed needle-wire system is available for breast lesion localization. After positioning of the needle tip in the proximity of the lesion, its stylet is removed and a flexible wire is inserted through the needle and advanced into the tissue adjacent to the lesion; the needle is immediately removed, leaving the wire in place. Frank and Hall[8] and Kopans and deLuca[20] have used a wire with a tip that bends back on itself. Once this flexible hook wire enters the breast parenchyma, it cannot be withdrawn easily because of its self-retaining character. If the wire is not properly placed, it can be extracted during localization or surgery by steady traction. Minor tissue damage along the wire tract can be expected as the hooked distal portion of the marker straightens. The straight end of the hook wire should be long enough to extend out beyond the skin surface. If the wire is inadvertently introduced into the underlying pectoralis musculature, its self-retaining feature may cause it to reposition into the breast with arm movement or other change in body position. In such circumstances, a hemostat placed on the outer end of the wire will prevent further internal migration of the wire. Taping the wire to the skin is unnecessary and will prevent motion of the wire during changes in patient position or breast compression. The skin area and exposed wire are covered with a sterile drape before the patient is transferred to surgery[13] (Fig 11–3).

Localization Using a Compression Plate With Perforations

A modified mammographic compression plate can be used for breast lesion localization. With this modification a compression plate is outfitted with a Plexiglas window regularly perforated with holes of a fixed diameter. The holes are marked in a coordinate system by engraved letters and numbers (Fig 11–4). In case of lesion localization or aspiration, the perforated plate is used instead of the usual compression plate.

The compression plate with the perforations should be placed as near as possible to the lesion. Ideally, the lesion should be situated under the center of the perforated compression plate. Therefore, lesions in the upper quadrants

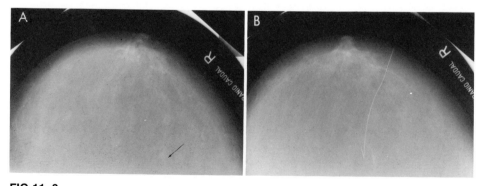

FIG 11–3.
A, a craniocaudal view shows a small nonpalpable mass *(arrow)*. **B,** a craniocaudal view shows the flexible hookwire adjacent to the suspicious mass.

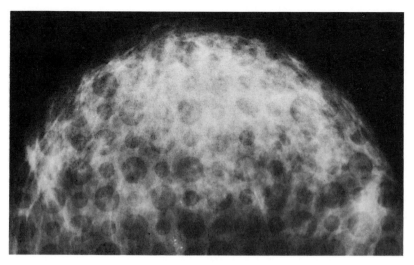

FIG 11–4.
Compression plate with perforations used for localization of breast lesions. (Courtesy of Siemens.)

are approached from the craniocaudal projection, those in the lower outer quadrant from the lateromedial projection, and those in the lower inner quadrant from the mediolateral oblique projection. The operator defines the positioning of the x-ray tube and compression plate on the basis of previous mammographic films. After the x-ray tube and perforated compression plate are adjusted, the breast is compressed and the film is exposed with the greatest possible distance between the film and the tube. The perforations are projected over the breast on the mammograms. The needle or hooked wire is then inserted through the hole under which the lesion is situated. Advancement of the needle should parallel the x-ray beam.[26, 32]

Fine-Needle Aspiration of Breast Cysts

Fibrocystic disease is one of the most common diseases of the breast. Additionally, patients with this diagnosis have a threefold increased risk of developing breast cancer.[34]

On mammography, benign cysts are round or ovoid and well-delineated and sometimes are surrounded by a thin radiolucent line. They are not associated with the classic signs of malignancy: irregular and ill-defined mass lesion, microcalcification, increased vascularity, and skin thickening and retraction. Malignant masses often appear larger by palpation than by mammography; this may be related to surrounding edema. Mammography offers the best means of diagnosis in breast disease, but the differential diagnosis between benign and malignant disease is not always possible.

Sonography is a highly reliable means for detection of small fluid-filled masses (Fig 11–5,A). Breast cysts are echo-free and demonstrate posterior through transmission with refractive shadowing behind the edges of the cyst.[18] They may have a small amount of internal echogenicity, due to the presence

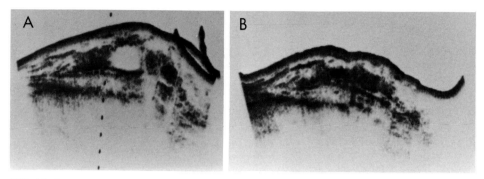

FIG 11–5.
A, transverse sonogram demonstrating a simple breast cyst. **B,** transverse sonogram following complete aspiration of cyst by a 22-gauge needle.

of debris or particulate matter within the cystic contents. Irregularity of the cyst wall or development of a mass in a cyst wall can be evaluated with ultrasound (US). Small cystic masses tend to be spherical; larger cysts tend to be more variable in shape owing to constraints from the surrounding tissues or to the presence of other lesions.

Aspiration of breast cysts can be performed[12] (Fig 11–5,B). When doing so, one must take care not to disregard the possibility of a carcinoma arising in or adjacent to the cyst.[24] The risk of this can be minimized by complete evacuation of the cyst and reexamination of the breast by mammography. The cyst fluid should be evaluated by cytology regardless of its appearance. Sonography can be used for localization for cyst aspiration. Any cystic mass that is suspicious for neoplasm on US but has negative cytologic aspirate should be biopsied surgically or closely observed.[33]

Pneumocystography

Pneumocystography is used to detect or rule out an intracystic tumor. The breast cyst is punctured and the fluid contents of the cyst are completely evaluated. Air is insufflated into the cyst and the needle is removed. Craniocaudal and mediolateral mammograms are taken to evaluate the inner structure of the cyst and the inner aspect of the cyst wall. An air-filled cyst is seen as a radiolucent mass with a thin, regular, and smooth wall. A thick and irregular wall is regarded as suspicious and indicates a need for open biopsy.[15]

It is recommended that pneumocystography be followed with mammography in approximately three months.[34] If there is no suspicion of an intracystic tumor and if cytologic examination of the aspirate is negative, operative removal of the cyst is unnecessary.

Fine-Needle Aspiration of Solid and Nonpalpable Masses

Aspiration biopsy can be utilized of all breast lesions. Cystic or solid, inflammatory or neoplastic lesions can be biopsied. Even nonpalpable lesions detected by mammography can be biopsied percutaneously. Localization can be accomplished by any of the previously described techniques. A 22-gauge needle is inserted into the lesion under aseptic conditions. Such a biopsy can yield a prompt diagnosis, allowing the physician to facilitate treatment planning and patient preparation. It is even possible to obtain a small core of solid breast tissue for histologic examination. Because it is an outpatient procedure, there can be financial benefits to this type of approach.

INVASIVE INTRAUTERINE TECHNIQUES

Amniocentesis

Amniocentesis is the primary diagnostic technique for prenatal diagnosis of genetic disorders such as cytogenetic abnormalities, metabolic diseases, neural tube defects, hemoglobinopathies, and x-linked traits.[3, 35] Guidance with US for amniocentesis results in a significant decrease in the number of attempts required, and a decrease in the number of bloody aspirations than when the procedure is performed blindly.[2, 25, 28] Ultrasound facilitates placental localization. Additionally, US provides an assessment of fetal viability and fetal morphology. The information obtained by prenatal US may also provide information that obviates the need for amniocentesis. Ultrasound aids in demonstrating twin gestational sacs and identifying the membrane between the two fetuses so that both sacs can be localized separately for amniocentesis.

Sonographically determined fetal age is valuable in determining the appropriate time for amniocentesis and also for correctly evaluating alpha-fetoprotein values or amniotic fluid volume. The amniotic fluid turnover is rapid and continuous. At 15 to 16 weeks gestational age, there are 150 to 200 ml of fluid in the amniotic sac, and the volume increases 50 ml per week for the next 13 weeks.[9] When gestational age is known, amniocentesis can be performed around 15 to 16 weeks, allowing sufficient time to repeat the procedure if cell culture fails.

Technique

All patients are examined for fetal number, fetal age, and placental position. The fetus should be carefully examined, including inspection of the head and intracranial contents, the spine, heart, kidneys, bladder, and extremities. The maternal heart rate is taken and recorded as a baseline and the patient empties her urinary bladder.

Emptying of the bladder allows the uterus to be in its normal position. A distended bladder can push and rotate the uterus, altering the position of the placenta in relation to the maternal midline. The chance of aspirating urine from the maternal urinary bladder instead of the amniotic cavity is decreased with voiding.

The site of entry into the amniotic cavity is determined by US. Ideally, the puncture site is located in the miduterine cavity anteriorly, away from both the fundus and lower uterine segment. An approach through the lateral aspect of the uterus should be avoided because of its typically high vascularity. The corresponding site of entry on the maternal abdomen is usually along the midabdominal line; however, on rare occasions, it may be slightly away from the midline because of tilting of the uterus to the right or left of the abdomen and pelvis. Localization of amniotic fluid is accomplished by B-mode or real-time sonography in two perpendicular planes. The angle of approach and depth from the skin to the amniotic cavity are determined from the scanner.

Needle insertion for amniocentesis can be performed with and without the use of a biopsy transducer. With accurate localization of the amniotic cavity, use of a biopsy transducer is not necessary. It does, however, allow monitoring the needle tip during advancement, thereby minimizing trauma to the fetus. After verifying the angle of approach, the needle is advanced in one smooth motion into the amniotic cavity to the previously determined depth from the skin. Advancement of the needle in one motion minimizes tenting of the membranes and deflection of the needle off the uterus. The stylet is then removed to check for flow of amniotic fluid. If fluid is not obtained, the stylet should be reinserted and the needle advanced to a greater depth or withdrawn to a more superficial position. Replacement of the needle stylet reduces the risk of contaminating the sample with maternal tissue. If amniotic fluid is not obtained a second needle should be used for the next attempt. Once the amniotic cavity is entered, gentle suction with a 10- or 20-ml syringe is used for aspiration of 20 to 25 ml of fluid, a volume sufficient for cell culture and analysis. Gentle traction minimizes contamination of the sampling with maternal cells.

In case of twin pregnancy the procedure is modified. After aspiration of amniotic fluid from the first sac, 0.5 ml of indigo carmine dye is injected before the needle is removed. This localizes the first sac that was sampled. Indigo carmine is used rather than methylene blue, as use of the latter has been associated with hemolytic anemia of the neonate.[6] The maternal abdomen is manually manipulated to distribute the dye and the second amniocentesis is performed. Aspiration of clear fluid indicates that the second sac has been entered.

In the situation of an anterior placenta, puncture of the main bulk of the placenta, the area of umbilical cord insertion, and the umbilical cord should be avoided.[16] If the placenta cannot be avoided, the shortest possible path through the placenta is selected (Fig 11–6). The amniotic fluid should be transported at room temperature to the laboratory in the original syringes or in sterile-treated glass or plastic tubes.

Causes of Failure

Improper placement of the needle and inadequate penetration of amniotic cavity are the major causes of failure of amniocentesis in our institution. There are at least three explanations for inadequate penetration of the needle. The patient may develop a myometrial contraction[7] during amniocentesis, so the distance between the maternal skin and amniotic cavity is increased. In such cases, both advancement and/or withdrawal of the needle are difficult and the procedure must be delayed until the contraction is resolved. The second possible cause of failure to enter the amniotic cavity is membrane tenting.[27] In this situation, the depth of the needle penetration is adequate, but the needle tip does not penetrate into the amniotic cavity. For puncture of the amniotic membrane in such circumstances, the needle is withdrawn and reinserted again with

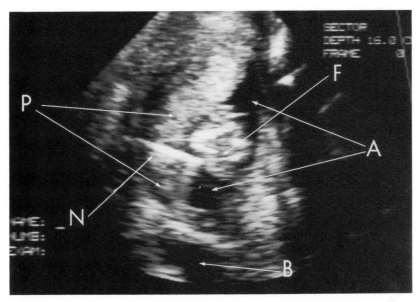

FIG 11–6.
Amniocentesis by a 22-gauge needle through an anterior placenta under guidance of real-time ultrasonography. *A* = amniotic fluid; *B* = bladder; *F* = fetus; *N* = needle.

a sharper motion. Inaccurate calibration of the scanner measurements can result in both under- and overestimation of the depth of the amniotic cavity from the skin.

Complications

The major complications associated with genetic amniocentesis are bloody fluid samples, spontaneous abortion, spontaneous rupture of membranes with leakage of amniotic fluid, infection, fetal trauma, maternal needle tract endometriosis, and maternal Rh-sensitization.[11, 22, 29]

A bloody tap may indicate damage to the fetus or placenta. Contamination of amniotic fluid by fetal blood results in significant elevation of the levels of alpha-fetoprotein, a protein found in high concentration in fetal serum. This can lead to problems in the assessment of a fetus at risk of developing a neural tube defect. The frequency of bloody samples as reported in isolated studies ranged from 55% to 22%.[10] The blood is almost always of maternal origin and apparently does not adversely affect amniotic cell growth.[35] The incidence of complicating spontaneous abortion has been reported from 0.6% to 7.5%. Since there is a definite risk of spontaneous abortion at this gestational age even when amniocentesis is not performed, the significance of these percentages is undetermined. Additionally, as the number of needle insertions increases, the frequency of rupture of membranes also increases from 0.9% to 3.6%.

The most common sign of fetal injury from amniocentesis is the presence of cutaneous scars, such as depressions or dimples, on the child.[10] The frequency has been reported to be 0.9% to 9.3%. The risk of musculoskeletal deformity and congenital dislocation of the hips is also increased following genetic amniocentesis. Musculoskeletal abnormalities occurred in 1% of maternal subjects as compared with 0.2% of controls. This abnormality may be attributed to a state of chronic oligohydramnios following amniocentesis.

Fetal Intervention

Percutaneous invasive procedures are being performed on human fetuses in the hope of arresting or reversing damage to fetal organs.[1, 14] With the advent of high-resolution US, it is now possible to clearly visualize the fetus in the uterine cavity. The internal organs such as the kidneys and bladder, and pathological processes such as ascites, can be easily demonstrated and localized. A hydronephrotic kidney or distended urinary bladder can be punctured under the direct monitoring of real-time US.

Percutaneous Needle Aspiration of the Fetal Bladder, Kidneys, Chest or Abdominal Cavities

Percutaneous fine-needle aspiration can be performed for diagnostic purposes or for treatment. With this technique, the size of the target, be it a hydronephrotic kidney, the urinary bladder, or ascites, is not as critical as it is for catheter insertion. No patient preparation is necessary except for premedication if desired. The procedure is similar to that of diagnostic amniocentesis. After preparation of the skin, a 22-gauge needle is inserted under direct monitoring by real-time US. The tip of the needle can be visualized in the desired location and can be confirmed by fluid aspiration (Fig 11–7).

With oligohydramnios, reduced fetal movement decreases the risks of fine-needle aspiration. With a normal amount of amniotic fluid, normal movement and reaction to the stimulation will increase the risk of traumatizing the fetus.

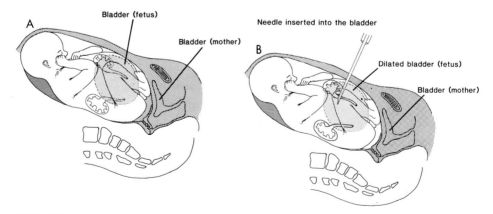

FIG 11–7.
A, a schematic drawing shows a fetus with distended bladder and hydronephrosis. **B,** following localization of the bladder, a 22-gauge needle is inserted into the bladder under continuous observation by real-time.

There are three possible ways to reduce the risk of fetal trauma. The mother can be sedated with morphine to decrease fetal activity. Alternatively, in certain instances, it may be possible to hold the fetus manually during the procedure. The procedure could also be performed with a fine-needle (22-gauge) fitted with a Teflon sheath. Following localization and puncture, the needle can be removed, leaving the Teflon sheath in place. The procedure should be performed in one quick motion, with the needle or sheath quickly removed after aspiration of fluid or urine.

In circumstances where there is bilateral hydronephrosis due to posterior urethral valves or bilateral obstruction of the ureteropelvic junction, repeated transabdominal aspirations may be performed, but they will obviously not result in permanent resolution of either condition.[21] The frequency of complications will increase in direct proportion to the number of aspirations. Repeated transabdominal aspirations are therefore not recommended unless performed over a short period of time. The procedure is recommended for diagnostic purposes, to attempt to prevent rupture of a hydronephrotic kidney, and to facilitate vaginal delivery. To avoid sudden alterations in fetal hemodynamics, the urine from these obstructed urinary tracts should be drained very slowly.[19]

REFERENCES

1. Berkowitz EL, et al: Fetal urinary tract obstruction: What is the role of surgical intervention in utero? *Am J Obstet Gynecol* 1982; 144:367–397.
2. Carpenter RJ, Hinkley CM, Carpenter AF: Midtrimester genetic amniocentesis: Use of ultrasound direction vs. blind needle insertion. *J Reprod Med* 1983; 28:35–40.
3. Cho S, et al: Prenatal diagnosis. *J Kansas Med Soc* 1981; 82:393–398.
4. Dodd GD, Fry K, Delany W: Preoperative localization of occult carcinoma of the breast, in Nealson TR (ed): *Management of the Patient With Cancer*. Philadelphia, WB Saunders Co, 1965, pp 88–113.
5. Eagan JF, Sayler CB, Goodman MJ: A technique for localizing occult breast lesions. *CA* 1976; 26:32–37.
6. Elias S, et al: Genetic amniocentesis in twin gestations. *Am J Obstet Gynecol* 1980; 158:169–174.
7. Finberg HG, Frigoletto FD: Sonographic demonstration of uterine contraction during amniocentesis. *Am J Obstet Gynecol* 1981; 139:740–742.
8. Frank HA, Hall FJ: Preoperative localization of nonpalpable breast lesions demonstrated by mammography. *N Engl J Med* 1976; 295:259–260.
9. Fuchs F: Volume of amniotic fluid at various stages of pregnancy. *Clin Obstet Gynecol* 1966; 9:449.
10. Galle PC, Meis PJ: Complications of amniocentesis: A review. *J Reprod Med* 1982; 27:149–155.
11. Golbus MS, et al: Rh isoimmunization following genetic amniocentesis. *Prenatal Diagn* 1982; 2:149–156.
12. Haagensen CD: Cystic disease of the breast, in Haagensen CD (ed): *Diseases of the Breast*. Philadelphia, WB Saunders Co, 1971, pp 155–176.
13. Hall FJ, Frank HA: Preoperative localization of nonpalpable breast lesions. *AJR* 1979; 132:101–105.

14. Harrison MR: Perinatal management of the fetus with a correctable defect, in *Ultrasonography in Obstetrics and Gynecology*. Philadelphia, WB Saunders Co, 1983, pp 177–192.

15. Hebert G, Ouimet-Oliva D: Diagnosis and management of cysts. *AJR* 1972; 115:801.

16. Hill JA, Reindollar RH, McDonough PG: Ultrasonic placental localization in relation to spontaneous abortion after mid-trimester amniocentesis. *Prenatal Diagn* 1982; 2:289–295.

17. Horns WJ, Arndt RD: Percutaneous spot localization of nonpalpable breast lesions. *AJR* 1976; 127:253–256.

18. Jellins J, Kossoff G, Reeve TS: Detection and classification of liquid-filled masses in the breast by gray-scale echography. *Radiology* 1977; 125:205–212.

19. Kirkinen P, et al: Repeated transabdominal renocenteses in a case of fetal hydronephrotic kidney. *Am J Obstet Gynecol* 1982; 142:1048–1052.

20. Kopans DB, de Luca S: A modified hook-wire technique to simplify preoperative localization of occult breast lesions. *Radiology* 1980; 134:781.

21. Kramer SA: Current status of fetal intervention of congenital hydronephrosis. *J Urol* 1983; 130:641–646.

22. Lele AS, et al: Fetomaternal bleeding following diagnostic amniocentesis. *Obstet Gynecol* 1982; 60:60–64.

23. Libshitz HI, Ferg SA, Fetouh S: Needle localization of nonpalpable breast lesions. *Radiology* 1976; 121:557–560.

24. McSwain GR, Valicenti JF, O'Brien PH: Cytologic evaluation of breast cysts. *Surg Gynecol Obstet* 1978; 146:921–925.

25. Mennuti MT, et al: Fetal-maternal bleeding associated with genetic amniocentesis: Real-time versus static ultrasound. *Obstet Gynecol* 1983; 62:26–30.

26. Muhlow A: A device for precision needle biopsy of the breast at mammography. *AJR* 1974; 121:843–845.

27. Platt LD, DeVore GR, Gimovsky ML: Failed amniocentesis: The role of membrane tenting. *Am J Gynecol* 1982; 144:479–480.

28. Porreco RP, et al: Reproductive outcome following amniocentesis for genetic indications. *Am J Obstet Gynecol* 1982; 148:653–660.

29. Romero R, et al: Antenatal sonographic diagnosis of umbilical cord laceration. *Am J Obstet Gynecol* 1982; 148:719–720.

30. Shepard D, et al: Mammography: An aid in the treatment of carcinoma of the breast. *Ann Surg* 1974; 179:749–755.

31. Simon N, et al: Roentgenographic localization of small lesions of the breast by the spot method. *Surg Gynecol Obstet* 1972; 134:572–574.

32. Tabar L, Dean PB: Interventional radiologic procedures in the investigation of lesions of the breast. *Radiol Clin North Am* 1979; 17:607–621.

33. Tabar L, Péntek Z: Pneumocystography of benign and malignant intracystic growths of the female breast. *Acta Radiol* 1975; 17:829–837.

34. Tabar L, Pénetek Z, Dean PB: The diagnostic and therapeutic value of breast cyst puncture and pneumocystography. *Radiology* 1981; 141:659–663.

35. Verp MS, Gerbie AB: Amniocentesis for prenatal diagnosis. *Clin Obstet Gynecol* 1981; 24:1007–1021.

Index

A

Abdomen (*See also* Intra-abdominal abscess; Transabdominal biopsy)
  fetal, 156
Abscess (*See also* Fluid collections)
  drainage of, 121–137 (*See also specific locations*)
    history of, 122–123
    imaging in, 123–125
    management in, 125–128
    puncture in, 125
    results of, 134–136
    techniques for, 123–125
    trocar technique in, 125
  hepatic, 107
    amebic, 129
    biopsy of, 105
    computed tomography of, 124
    drainage of, 111–117, 128–130
    pyogenic, 129–130
  iliopsoas, drainage of, 143
  intra-abdominal, drainage of, 130–131
  intraloop
    drainage of, 131
    ultrasonography of, 123
  pancreatic
    definition of, 132
    diagnostic aspiration of, 74–76
    drainage of, 76, 132–134
    localization of, 71–73
    multiloculated, 73
    multiple, 73
  pelvic
    drainage of, 131–132
    ultrasonography of, 123
  perinephric, 96–97, 99
  pulmonary
    parenchymal, computed tomography of, 56
    ultrasonography of, 42
  renal, 89–91
    diagnostic aspiration of, 90
    predisposing factors in, 89
    technique for aspiration and drainage of, 91
    therapeutic aspiration of, 90, 99
  subphrenic
    computed tomography of, 124
    drainage of, 130–131
  thoracic, irrigation of, 56
Accordion catheter, 22–23, 25
Accuracy rate
  of fine-needle aspiration biopsy, 1
  of liver biopsy, 105
  of pancreatic biopsy, 63
  of percutaneous adrenal biopsy, 96
  of transthoracic needle aspiration, computed tomography guided, 55
  of ultrasonography
    in hepatic lesions, 112
    in renal cysts, 81
Acoustic coupling agents, 6
Adenocarcinoma, pancreatic
  biopsy of, 66
  ultrasonography of, 67

Adrenal gland
 biopsy of, 95–96
  diagnostic yield and accuracy of, 96
 puncture of, in renal biopsy, 95
Air embolism, lung biopsy causing, 36
Alcohol, renal cyst sclerosis with, 89
All-purpose Drainage Catheter, 23
Amebic liver abscess, 107
Amniocentesis, 153–156
 complications of, 155–156
 failure of, 154–155
 technique of, 153–154
Amplatz needle, 19, 26
Aneurysm, false, in renal biopsy, 95
Angiography, 60 (*See also* Seldinger
  technique)
 in cystic renal masses, 80, 81
 in pancreatic biopsy, 63
 in pancreatic localization, 67
 in urinary tract, 64
Antegrade pyelography, 60, 64
Antibacterial medication, for hepatic abscess, 113
Antibiotics
 before biopsy or drainage, 12
 following pancreatic biopsy, 71
Antiparasitic medication, for hepatic abscess, 113
Aortography needle, translumbar, 19,
  26
Arteriotomy needle, Amplatz, 26
Arteriovenous fistula
 in renal biopsy, 95
 in renal cyst puncture, 87
Ascites, perihepatic, 117
Aspirate (*see* Specimen)
Aspiration biopsy
 accuracy rate of, 1
 contraindications to, 13
 dry vs. wet, 16
 general considerations in, 1
 general technique for, 11–16
Aspiration drainage, 1 (*See also specific
  locations*)
Atelectasis, ultrasonography of, 46
Attenuation value, of renal cysts, interiors of, 81
Auger biopsy, biliary, 108

B

Bacteriologic examination, needles for,
  8
Barium, opacification with, duodenal
  loop, 63
Bile duct(s)
 common, cholangiography of, 63

 dilatation of, 67
 hepatic cyst rupture into, 109
 obstruction of, 107
Biliary biopsy, 107–108
Biliary diversion, percutaneous, 116
Biloma, 117
 traumatic, hepatic abscess vs., 112
Biopsy notch, 15
Biopsy window, 9
Biplane fluoroscopy
 of retroperitoneal masses, 60
 technique of, 62
 transthoracic, 31
Bladder
 fetal, 156
 neurogenic, renal abscess and, 89
Bleeding (*See also* Hemorrhage)
 as lung biopsy contraindication, 37
"Blind" liver biopsy, 104
Blood urea nitrogen, 12
B-mode scanning
 in pancreatic biopsy, 69–70
 in pleural effusion, 44
Bowel, puncture of, in renal biopsy, 95
Breast
 fibrocystic disease of, aspiration of,
  151–152
 masses of
  aspiration of, 152–153
  biopsy of, 146–153
  needle localization of, 149
  nonpalpable, localization of, 146
  perforated compression plate localization of, 150–151
  self-retaining wire localization of,
   150
  spot method localization of,
   146–147
  surface method localization of, 146
 pneumocystography of, 152
Bronchial tree, thoracic abscess and, 57
Brush biopsy, biliary, 107

C

Cancer (*See also* Tumors)
 pancreatic
  diagnosis of, 67
  fluoroscopy-guided biopsy of, 63
C-arm fluoroscopy
 of retroperitoneal masses, 60
 technique of, 62
 in transthoracic biopsy, 31
Catheter(s)
 accordion, 25
  Hawkins, 22–23
 All-purpose Drainage, 23

C-flex drainage, 24
  McLean sump, 24
  multiple, in hepatic abscess drainage, 116
  sump, 24
    in hepatic abscess drainage, 116
    vanSonnenberg, 23–24
Catheter drainage, 1, 21–26 *(See also specific locations)*
  biliary, 108
  of pancreatic abscess or pseudocyst, 76
  Seldinger technique of, 24–26 *(See also* Seldinger technique*)*
  trocar technique of, 21–24 *(See also* Trocar technique*)*
Cavernous hemangioma, 107
CBC count, 12
  before transthoracic biopsy, 32
Cell block examination, 19
Cellular examination, 16–18
C-flex drainage catheter, 24
Chest
  fetal, 156
  masses of, biopsy of, fluoroscopy-guided, 30–38 *(See also* Transthoracic biopsy*)*
  ultrasonography of, 40
Chiba needle, 8
  transabdominal biopsy with, 60
  transthoracic biopsy with, 32, 33
Cholangiocarcinoma, 107
Cholangiography
  of common bile duct, 63
  in pancreatic localization, 67
  percutaneous, 60
  transhepatic
    of abscess, 112
    of biliary lesions, 108
Cholangiopancreatography, retrograde, endoscopic, 60
  in pancreatic biopsy, 63
  in pancreatic cancer diagnosis, 67
  in pancreatic pseudocyst, 73
Coaxial technique, 8, 14
  hepatic, 107
  modified *(see* Modified coaxial technique*)*
  needle placement in, in pancreatic biopsy, 70
  transabdominal, fluoroscopy-guided, 62
  transthoracic, 34–35
    computed tomography guided, 53–55
Complete blood cell (CBC) count, 12
  before transthoracic biopsy, 32

Computed tomography, 2, 20, 21
  in abscess drainage, 123–125
  in kidney
    abscess aspiration and drainage of, 91
    cystic masses of, 80–81
      aspiration of, 85
  in liver
    abscess of, 111–112
      drainage of, 115
    biopsy of, 104–105
    cyst of, 109–111
    focal masses of, 105
    neoplastic and inflammatory disease of, 107
    solid masses of, 107
  localization with, 6–8
  in pancreas, 66–76
    abscess of, 73
    aspiration of, 74
    biopsy of, 63
    fluid collections in, 71–72
    fluoroscopy vs., 68
    masses of, 67
    ultrasonography vs., 68
      masses in, 67
  transabdominal, fluoroscopy vs., 60
  transthoracic
    aspiration in, 55
    drainage of fluid collections in, 55–57
      results of, 57
    fluoroscopy vs., 51–52
    lung lesions in, 31
    masses in, 51–57
      patient position for, 53
Contrast, with computed tomography localization, 12
Contrast enhancement, of renal cysts, 81
Contrast medium
  extravasation of, in renal cyst puncture, 87
  sensitivity to, renal cyst aspiration and, 85
Cope single-stick system, 24–25 *(See also* Single-stick technique*)*
Cradle-top table, rotational, in transabdominal fluoroscopy, 60
Creatinine, 12
CT *(see* Computed tomography*)*
Cutaneous seeding, pancreatic biopsy causing, 71
Cutting needles, 8–9
  technique with, 14–15
  in transthoracic biopsy, 34
Cyst(s)
  breast, aspiration of, 151–152

Cyst(s) *(cont.)*
  echinococcal, 13
    hepatic abscess vs., 112
    risk in biopsy of, 107
  hepatic *(see* Hepatic cysts)
  infected, hepatic abscess vs., 112
  pulmonary, ultrasonography of, 42
  puncture of, with cystogram, 80
  renal *(see* Renal cysts)
Cystadenocarcinoma, diagnosis of, 72
Cystadenoma, diagnosis of, 72
Cystogram
  cyst puncture with, 80
  patient position for, 87
  technique of, 85–87
Cytogenetic abnormalities, 153
Cytologic examination, 1, 18–19
  needles for, 8
  pancreatic, cancer diagnosis and, 67
  of retroperitoneal biopsy specimen, 63

D

Density, of renal cysts, on computed to-
    mography, 82
Diabetes, renal abscess and, 89
Diaphragm, localization of, ultrasonog-
    raphy in, 42
Dionosil, for sinograms, 57
Double-contrast study, of renal cyst, 87
Dry aspiration, 16
Duodenal loop, barium opacification of,
    63
Dynamic scanning, in pancreatic biopsy,
    70

E

Echinococcal cysts, 13
  hepatic abscess vs., 112
  risk in biopsy of, 107
Effusion, pleural *(see* Pleural effusion)
Electronic marking line, 2
Embolism, air, lung biopsy causing, 36
Emphysema, lung biopsy causing, 37
Empyema, drainage of
  computed tomography guided, 57
  ultrasonography guided, 42, 46
Endoscopic retrograde cholangiopan-
    creatography, 60
  in pancreatic biopsy, 63
  in pancreatic cancer diagnosis, 67
  in pancreatic pseudocyst, 73
Enteric fistula, drainage of, 131
Enteric leak, 131, 136
Ethanol fixation, 19

Excretory pyelography, 60
Extravasation, of contrast medium, in
    renal cyst puncture, 87

F

Fasting, in patient preparation, 11–12
  for transthoracic biopsy, 32
Fetus *(See also* Amniocentesis)
  intervention with, 156–157
Fever, in renal cyst puncture, 87
Fibrocystic disease, breast, aspiration of,
    151–152
Fine-needle aspiration *(See* Aspiration
    biopsy: *specific locations)*
Fistula
  arteriovenous
    in renal biopsy, 95
    in renal cyst puncture, 87
  controlled, 131
  enteric, drainage of, 131
  formation of, pancreatic biopsy caus-
      ing, 66, 70
Fluid, in hepatic cysts, 109
Fluid collections *(See also* Abscess; *specific
    locations)*
  drainage of, 19–26
    instrumentation for, 19–20
  perihepatic, 117
  perinephric, 96–99
    diagnostic and therapeutic aspira-
        tion of, 99
    localization of, 99
  simple aspiration of, 19
Fluoroscopy, 2, 20, 21
  in biopsy of chest masses, 30–38 *(See
      also* Transthoracic biopsy)
  computed tomography vs., 51–52
    in pancreas, 68
    transabdominal, 60
  in localization of lung lesions, 31
  lymph node, 64
    pelvic, 142
  in renal abscess aspiration and drain-
      age, 91
  in renal cyst aspiration, 82–85
  in renal mass aspiration, solid, 91
  in transabdominal biopsy of retroperi-
      toneal masses, 59–64
    technique of, 60–63
  ultrasonography vs., in renal cyst aspi-
      ration, 85
  in urinary tract, 64
Franseen needle, 9
  in transabdominal biopsy, 60–61
  in transthoracic biopsy, 32
Furuncles, skin, renal abscess and, 89

G

Gallbladder
  intrahepatic, hepatic abscess vs., 112
  perforation of, renal biopsy causing,
    95
Gallium scanning, of hepatic abscess,
  129
Gas
  in hepatic abscess, 112
  in pancreatic fluid collections, 72–73
Gram-negative organisms, renal abscess
  and, 89
Greene biopsy set, 9
Greene needle, 8–9
  in transabdominal biopsy, 60
  in transthoracic biopsy, 32
Grid, in computed tomography, 7
  of thoracic fluid collections, 56
Guidewire biopsy, biliary, 108

H

Hawkins accordion catheter, 22–23
Hawkins single-stick system, 25
Hemangioma, cavernous, 107
Hematoma
  hepatic abscess vs., 112
  pancreatic, diagnosis of, 72
  perihepatic, 117
  perinephric, 96, 97–98, 99
  pleural, ultrasonography of, 42
  renal, therapeutic aspiration of, 99
  renal biopsy causing, 95
Hematuria
  in renal biopsy, 95
  renal cyst puncture causing, 87
Hemithorax, loculated pleural effusions
  in, ultrasonography of, 42
Hemoglobinopathies, 153
Hemoptysis
  lung biopsy causing, 36
  thoracic aspiration causing, 48
Hemorrhage
  hepatic cyst and, 109
  lung biopsy causing, 36
  pancreatic biopsy causing, 66, 70
  pancreatic pseudocyst causing, 73–74
  perirenal, renal cyst puncture causing,
    87
  polycystic liver disease and, 111
Hemorrhagic pancreatitis, abscess in, 72
Hepatic abnormalities, focal, 104
Hepatic abscess
  amebic, 129
  computed tomography of, 124
  drainage of, 111–117, 128–130

  failure rate in, 116
  pyogenic, 129–130
    hepatic cyst vs., 112
  success rate in, 116
Hepatic cysts
  biopsy of, 108–111
  communication of, with vascular or
    biliary structures, 111
  complications of, 109
  congenital, 109
  differential diagnosis of, 111
  hepatic abscess vs., 112
Hepatic disease, liver biopsy in, 104
Hepatic fluid collections, 112
Hepatic mass
  benign, biopsy of, 105
  focal, biopsy of, 105–111
  solid or complex, 106–108
Hepatoblastoma, 107
Hepatoma, biopsy of, 106–108
Histologic examination, 1
Hydronephrosis, benign renal cyst causing, 88
Hypertension
  benign renal cyst causing, 88
  pulmonary, as lung biopsy contraindi-
    cation, 37

I

Iliac lymph node, lymphangiography of,
  64
Iliopsoas abscess, drainage of, 143
Image intensification, in lung nodule biopsy, 31
Imaging (*See also specific types*)
  in abscess drainage, 124–125
Infarction, lung, ultrasonography of, 46
Infection
  hepatic cyst and, 109
  pancreatic pseudocyst causing, 73
  polycystic liver disease and, 111
  renal cyst puncture causing, 87
Inflammatory lesions, hepatic, 107
Instrumentation, for aspiration biopsy,
  8–10
Intra-abdominal abscess, drainage of,
  130–131
Intrauterine techniques, 153–157
Intravenous pyelography (*see* Pyelography)
Iophendylate
  in hepatic cyst sclerosis, 111
  in renal cyst sclerosis, 88–89
Irrigation, of thoracic abscess, 56
Islet cell neoplasms, localization of, 67

K

Kidney *(See also* Renal *entries)*
  fetal, 156

L

Laboratory examination, 16–19
  before aspiration biopsy, 12
    transthoracic, 32
Lee needle, 9
  for transthoracic biopsy, 32
Lesions *(see* Masses)
Linear-array scanning, 2, 4
  of pleural effusion, 44
  renal, 85
Liver *(See also* Hepatic *entries)*
  biopsy of, 104–111
    indications for, 104
  diffuse parenchymal disease of, 104
    biopsy in, 105
  laceration of, renal biopsy causing, 95
Liver disease, polycystic, 111
Localization *(See also specific sites)*
  computed tomography, 6–8
  of fluid collections, 1, 2–6, 20
  of masses, 1, 2–6
Lung *(see* Pulmonary *entries:* Transthoracic biopsy)
Lymphangiography, 60
  in lymph node biopsy, 64
Lymphatic leakage, in lymphocele, 98
Lymph node biopsy, lymphangiography in, 64
Lymph nodes, pelvic, biopsy of, 140
  fluoroscopy in, 142
Lymphocele
  incidence of, 98
  pelvic, drainage of, 143
  perinephric, 96, 98–99
  therapeutic aspiration of, 99

M

McLean sump catheter, 24
Malignancy
  lung, thoracic aspiration causing, 49
  pancreatic, biopsy, risk in, 71
Marking line, electronic, 2
Masses
  adrenal, 96
  breast, 146–153 *(See also* Breast)
  hepatic, 105–108 *(See also* Hepatic mass)
  hilar, computed tomography of, 52
  localization of, 1 *(See also specific sites)*
  mediastinal, 52, 53, 55
  pancreatic, 66–71 *(See also* Pancreas)

pelvic, 139–144 *(See also* Pelvis)
perihilar, computed tomography of, 52
pleural-based, ultrasonography of, 46
pulmonary *(See* Pulmonary mass)
renal
  cystic *(see* Renal cysts)
  solid, 91
retroperitoneal, 59–64 *(See also* Retroperitoneum)
thoracic, 51–57 *(See also* Transthoracic biopsy)
Membrane filtration technique, 19
Menghini liver biopsy, 104
Metabolic diseases, 153
Metastases
  adrenal, 96
  hepatic, 107
Microabscess, hepatic, 129–130
Microbiologic examination, 18
Microhematuria, renal cyst puncture causing, 87
Mitty-Pollack needle, 19, 25
Modified coaxial technique, 8, 14
  transabdominal, fluoroscopy-guided, 62
  transthoracic, 34–35, 53–55

N

Necrotic neoplasms, hepatic abscess vs., 112
Necrotizing pancreatitis, abscess in, 72
Needle placement
  in pancreatic biopsy, 70
  transabdominal, fluoroscopy guided, 62
Needles *(See also specific needles)*
  aspiration, 8
  biopsy, 8–10
  cutting, 8–9
  for perinephric fluid collection aspiration, 99
  screw-type, 8, 10
  for transabdominal biopsy, 60–62
  translumbar aortography, 19, 26
  for transthoracic biopsy, 2
Needle-sheath system, in hepatic abscess drainage, 116
Needle size, and pancreatic biopsy complications, 70–71
Neoplasms *(see* Masses)
Nephrostomy needle, 26
Nephrotomography
  renal abscess in, 90
  renal mass detection with, 79
Neural tube defects, 153

Neurogenic bladder, renal abscess and, 89
Nodules, adrenal, nonfunctioning, benign, 96

O

Oligohydramnios, 156
One-Step Insertion needle, 25–26
Outpatient treatment, transabdominal biopsy, 61

P

Pain
  in renal cyst puncture, 87
  transthoracic aspiration causing, 48
Pancreas
  abscess of
    definition of, 132
    diagnostic aspiration of, 74–76
    drainage of, 76, 132–134
    localization of, 71–73
  adenocarcinoma of, 66–67
  biopsy of
    complications of, 70–71
    fluoroscopy-guided, 63
    intraoperative, complications of, 66–67
    localization in, 67–68
    technique for, 68–70
  cancer of, diagnosis of, 67
  computed tomography of, 66–76
  fluid collections in, drainage of, 132–134
    aspiration and, 71–76
  masses of, biopsy of, 66–71
  pseudocyst of (*see* Pseudocyst)
  puncture of, renal biopsy and, 95
  ultrasonography of, 66–76
Pancreatic duct, dilatation of, 67–68
Pancreatitis
  hemorrhagic, abscess in, 72
  necrotizing
    abscess in, 72
    fulminant, aspiration biopsy causing, 63
  pancreatic biopsy causing, 66, 70
Pantopaque (iophendylate)
  in hepatic cyst sclerosis, 111
  in renal cyst sclerosis, 88–89
Papanicolaou examination, of transabdominal specimen, 63
Partial thromboplastin time, 12
  before transthoracic biopsy, 32
Pelvis
  abscess of

drainage of, 131–132
ultrasonography of, 123
  fluid collections in, drainage of, 140
  lymphocele of, drainage of, 143
  masses of, 139–144
    biopsy of, 140
      complications of, 144
      results of, 140–144
    localization of, 139–140
Percu-flex, 23
Peritoneal cavity, free, hepatic cysts and, 109
Peritonitis, after pancreatic biopsy, 71
Phased-array real-time scanning, 5–6
Platelet count, 12
  before transthoracic biopsy, 32
Pleura
  mass of
    needles for biopsy of, 55
    ultrasonography of, 46
  ultrasonography of, 40
Pleural effusion
  diagnostic aspiration of, 45–46
  loculated, ultrasonography of, 42
  nonloculated, ultrasonography of, 41–42
  subpulmonary, ultrasonography of, 41
  ultrasonography of, 41–46
Pleural fluid collections, computed tomography of, 56
Pleural space
  computed tomography of, 53
  ultrasonography of, 40
Pneumocystography, breast, 152
Pneumonia, ultrasonography in, 46
Pneumothorax
  renal cyst puncture causing, 87
  after transthoracic biopsy, 33, 36–37, 55, 95
Polycystic liver disease, 111
Polycythemia, benign renal cysts causing, 88
Pregnancy, renal abscess and, 89
Premedication, 12
  for transabdominal biopsy, 61
Prostatism, renal abscess and, 89
Prothrombin time, 12
  before transthoracic biopsy, 32
Pseudocyst, pancreatic
  complications of, 73–74
  definition of, 132
  diagnostic aspiration of, 74–76
  drainage of, 76, 124, 134
  infected, 132
  localization of, 71, 73–74
  spontaneous regression of, 74
Pulmonary disease, infectious, 36

Pulmonary hypertension, as lung biopsy
  contraindication, 37
Pulmonary mass
  aspiration of
    results of, 48–49
    technique for, 47
    ultrasonography in, 46
  localization of, three-dimensional, 31
  peripheral, ultrasonography of, 46
Puncture
  in abscess drainage, 125
  for thoracentesis, 44
Pyelography, 60, 64
  in renal abscess, 90
    aspiration follow-up for, 91
Pyogenic liver abscess, 107

R

Radionuclide scanning
  of cystic renal masses, 80
  of hepatic abscess, 112, 129
Real-time scanning, 2, 5–6
  of focal hepatic masses, 105
  of pleural effusion, 44
  renal, 85
Renal abscess, 89–91
  aspiration of
    diagnostic and therapeutic, 90
    drainage and, technique of, 91
    therapeutic, 90, 99
  predisposing factors in, 89
Renal cysts
  analysis of aspirate from, 87
  aspiration of, 82–88
    complications of, 87–88
    computed tomography guided, 85
    fluoroscopy-guided, 82–85
    technique of, 85–87
    ultrasonography guided, 85
  diagnostic approach to, 79–82
    angiography in, 81
    computed tomography in, 81
    ultrasonography in, 80–81
  puncture of, complications of, 87–88
  slcerosis of, 88–89
Renal hematoma, therapeutic aspiration
  of, 99
Renal mass, solid, 91
Retrograde pyelography, 64
Retroperitoneum
  lymph nodes of, lymphangiography
    of, 64
  mass of
    localization of, 59–60
    transabdominal biopsy of, fluoros-
      copy-guided, 59–64

contraindications to, 63
  special considerations in, 63–64
  technique in, 60–63
Ribs, ultrasonographic interference of,
  41
Rotex biopsy instrument, 10
  technique with, 15–16
  transabdominal biopsy with, 60
  transthoracic biopsy with, 32, 34
Rupture
  hepatic cyst, 109
  pancreatic pseudocyst causing, 73

S

Scintigraphy (*see* Radionuclide scanning)
Sclerosis
  of hepatic cysts, 111
  of renal cysts, benign, 88–89
Screw-type biopsy instrument, Rotex (*see*
  Rotex biopsy instrument)
Screw-type needles, 8, 10
Sector real-time scanning, 2, 5–6
  of focal hepatic masses, 105
  of pleural effusion, 44
  renal, 85
  side-arm attachments in, 5–6
Seldinger technique, 24–26
  in hepatic abscess drainage, 116
  in lymphocele, 99
  in pancreatic abscess or pseudocyst
    drainage, 76
  in renal abscess, 99
    aspiration and drainage of, 91
  in renal hematoma, 99
  in transthoracic fluid collection drain-
    age, 56
  in urinoma, 99
Side-arm attachment
  for biopsy transducer, 4
  in renal aspiration, 85
  for sector scanners, 5–6
Simple aspiration biopsy, 14
Single-stick Seldinger technique, 24–26
  (*See also* Seldinger technique)
Sinography, in abscess drainage, 126
Skin furuncles, renal abscess and, 89
Specimen
  benign renal cyst, features of, 87
  cellular analysis of, 16–18
  chemical analysis of, 16–18
  cytologic analysis of, 18–19
  laboratory analysis of, 16–19
  microbiologic analysis of, 18
  transabdominal, cytologic analysis of,
    63

Spleen, laceration of, renal biopsy causing, 95
Staphylococci, renal abscess and, 89
Static scanners, 2
in pleural effusion, 44
Subphrenic abscess, computed tomography of, 124
Subphrenic fluid collections, ultrasonography of, 123
Subpleural space
computed tomography in, 53, 56
fluid collections in, 56
ultrasonography in, 40
Sump catheters, in hepatic abscess
drainage, 116 (*See also* Catheter;
Catheter drainage)
Sure-cut needle, 9
transabdominal biopsy with, 60
transthoracic biopsy with, 32
Syringe, dry, for transthoracic biopsy,
33

T

Table, cradle-top, rotational, in transabdominal fluoroscopy, 60
Tandem technique, 8, 14
in liver lesions, 107
in pancreatic abscess or pseudocyst
drainage, 76
in pancreatic biopsy, 70
in transabdominal biopsy, 62
in transthoracic biopsy, 34
Thoracentesis
puncture site for, 44
ultrasonography in, 42–46
Thoracic biopsy (*see* Transthoracic biopsy)
Tomography (*see* Computed tomography; Nephrotomography)
Transabdominal biopsy, fluoroscopy-
guided, of retroperitoneal masses,
59–64
contraindications to, 63
special considerations in, 63
technique of, 60–63
Transducers, 2–5
linear-array, 4
pancreatic scanning with, 69–70
real-time sector, 5–6
in renal aspiration, 85
side-arm attachment for, 4
Transhepatic cholangiography
in pancreatic biopsy, 63
pancreatic localization with, 67
percutaneous, of biliary lesions, 108

Translumbar aortography needle, 19,
26
Transthoracic biopsy, 30–38
abscess in
irrigation of, 56–57
ultrasonography of, 42
complications of, 36–37
with aspiration, 48–49
computed tomography guided, 55
contraindications to, 37
cyst in, ultrasonography of, 42
fluid collections in, drainage of, 55–57
general considerations in, 32–33
malignancy in, 35
masses in, 40–49
aspiration of, 47–49
complex, computed tomography of,
51–55
computed tomography of, 51–57
localization of, 51–55
solid, computed tomography of,
51–55
ultrasonography of, 42, 46
needles for, 32
patient preparation for, 32–33
results of, 35–36
specificity of, 35
specific techniques for, 33–35
ultrasonography in, normal lung in,
40–41
Trauma, pseudocyst and, 73
Trocar technique, 21–24
in abscess drainage, 125
in transthoracic fluid drainage, 56
Tru-cut needle, 9
in renal parenchymal disease, 95
in transthoracic biopsy, 32
Tumors (*See also* Masses)
hepatic, primary, 106–108
implantation of, lung biopsy causing,
36
islet cell, localization of, 67
lung, ultrasonography of, 42
Tumor seeding
in pancreas, 63, 71
pancreatic biopsy causing, 66
Turner needle, 8
transabdominal biopsy with, 60
transthoracic biopsy with, 32–34
Two-stick Seldinger technique, 26 (*See
also* Seldinger technique)

U

Ultrasonography, 1, 2, 8, 20, 21
in abscess drainage, 123

Ultrasonography *(cont.)*
  of chest, 40
  computed tomography vs., 51
    in pancreas, 67, 68
  in empyema drainage, 46
  fluoroscopy vs., in renal cyst aspiration, 85
  of hepatic abscess, 111–112
    drainage in, 115
  in hepatic biopsy, 104–105
  of hepatic cyst, 109–111
  of hepatic mass
    focal, 105
    solid, 106–107
  of lung, normal, 40–41
  of pancreas, 66–76
    aspiration in, 74
    biopsy in, 63
    computed tomography vs., 67, 68
    fluid collections in, 71
    intraoperative, 68
    masses in, 67
  in renal abscess aspiration and drainage, 91
  of renal masses
    cystic, 79
      aspiration in, 85
      diagnosis in, 80–82
    solid, aspiration in, 91
  in thoracentesis, 42–46
  thoracic, 40–49
    mass in, 46

Urinary tract, fluoroscopy of, 64
Urinoma
  perinephric, 96, 98, 99
  renal biopsy causing, 95
  renal cyst puncture causing, 87
  therapeutic aspiration of, 99
Urography, intravenous, renal mass detection with, 79

V

VanSonnenberg biopsy set, 9–10
VanSonnenberg sump catheter, 23–24
Vascular lesions, transabdominal biopsy of, fluoroscopy-guided, 63
Vascular structures, thoracic, computed tomography of, 52
Vim-Silverman needle, pancreatic biopsy with, 66
Volume averaging, partial, in renal cysts, 81

W

Westcott needle, 9
  for transthoracic biopsy, 32
Wet aspiration, 16

X

X-linked traits, 153